**Wygge.**  ᵗ h )

What You Need to Know About Cancer

# What You Need to Know About Cancer

• • •

## SCIENTIFIC AMERICAN
## A SPECIAL ISSUE

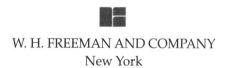

W. H. FREEMAN AND COMPANY
New York

Cover Design: Dorothy Wachtenheim/Victoria Tomaselli

Photographer, Science Source/Photo Researchers


**Library of Congress Cataloging-in-Publication Data**

What you need to know about cancer.
p.      cm.
"Scientific American, a special issue."
Includes bibliograpical references and index.
ISBN 0-7167-3102-9 (soft cover)
1. Cancer—Popular works.      I. Scientific American, Inc.
RC263.W464      1997
616.99'4—dc21                                                                            97-3663
                                                                                          CIP

The information in this book originally appeared in the September 1996 issue of Scientific American.

Printed in the United States of America

First printing 1997,  RRD

# Contents

· · ·

# What You Need to Know About Cancer

# Introduction:
# Making Headway against Cancer

*A single cure is still elusive, but for people touched by this disease,*
*modern understanding is paying off in better treatments,*
*better prevention and brighter prospects.*

• • •

John Rennie and Ricki Rusting

When President Richard M. Nixon signed the National Cancer Act two days before Christmas in 1971, he committed the United States to a "war" on cancer. In the 25 years since then, the battle has been waged around the world in laboratories, in hospitals, in our own homes and bodies. All of us are deluged with reports of scientific progress—dispatches from the front, so to speak—recounting incremental discoveries here, larger ones there, and widely hailed "breakthroughs" that translate into practice with frustrating rarity. Warnings about carcinogenic hazards blare one week, then get replaced by new advice that sometimes seems to conflict with what has already been said.

What, in fact, has medical science learned about cancer in the past quarter century? What real weapons do we now have for battling this foe, and what do all the miscellaneous discoveries mean for a worried public?

There is no way to skirt the fact that the combined death rate for all cancers has yet to come down. Indeed, between 1973 and 1992, the latest year for which comprehensive data are available, the cancer death rate rose by 6.3 percent. (This rate is measured as the number of people dying per 100,000 in the population and is "age-adjusted"—a maneuver that corrects for progress against other diseases and the rising longevity of the population.) African-Americans and people older than 65 years have fared particularly poorly; in both groups the overall death rate jumped by about 16 percent.

Epidemiologists projected that in 1996 nearly 555,000 U.S. cancer patients would die—up from 331,000 deaths in 1970. Some 40 percent of Americans will eventually be stricken with the disease, and more than one in five will die of it; the trends are broadly similar for most developed nations. Globally, the World Health Organization estimates that cancer kills roughly six million people annually.

But those forbidding statistics should not overshadow the equally real, galvanizing successes. For example, there have been striking reductions in death from some cancers, specifically Hodgkin's disease, Burkitt's lymphoma, testicular cancer, certain cancers of the bones and muscles, and a variety of malignancies that afflict children. The American Cancer Society reports that since 1960 the death rate from cancer in children has plummeted 62 percent.

The death toll from some of the greatest killers has begun to come down as well, at least for some segments of the population. Lung cancer mortality rates in men dropped by 3 percent between 1990 and 1992, largely from a decline in cigarette smoking over the past few decades. Breast cancer mortality rates fell by more than 5 percent between 1989 and 1993, most markedly in women younger than 65 and in whites. The decline appears to stem from a combination of early detection and, probably, improvements in treatment. And mortality from colorectal cancer fell by about 17 percent between 1973 and 1992, thanks to early detection and revised treatment strategies.

In fact, a close look at the mortality data (see the graph "Trends in U.S. Cancer Mortality from 1973 to 1992") reveals much cause for guarded optimism. The horrendous casualties from lung cancer obscure the general headway that has been made. Put aside lung cancer (a largely preventable disease), and the death rate from all other types has declined by 3.4 percent since 1973—by 13.3 percent in people younger than 65.

Much of this success derives, as Samuel Hellman and Everett E. Vokes of the University of Chicago describe in Chapter 8, "Advancing Current Treatments for Cancer," from new modes of therapy and more effective combinations and schedules of treatment. Therapeutic advances also include greater use of organ-sparing surgeries (which minimize disfigurement, pain and loss of function) and improvement in easing the side effects of therapy. Better attention is also paid to the emotional issues raised by the diagnosis and treatment of cancer. In short, a verdict of cancer does not necessarily carry the same bleak sentence it once did.

Certainly more needs to be done. Prevention is still an idea with plenty of untapped potential. An astonishing 30 percent of fatal cancers can be blamed primarily on smoking, and an equal number on lifestyle, especially dietary practices and lack of exercise. (One researcher has quipped that the best way to avoid cancer is to run from salad bar to salad bar.) By some estimates, if the govern-

ment, other authorities and individuals did more to reform risky behaviors, upward of 200,000 lives could be saved from cancer annually even if no new treatments were discovered.

More lives should also be spared as a result of the avalanche of fundamental findings about how cancer develops and progresses. That knowledge, hard won over the past 20 years, is providing the blueprints for totally new therapies that will exploit the characteristic molecular abnormalities of cancer cells.

Unfortunately, political and economic hurdles stand in the way of doing more to prevent cancer and threaten research aimed at improving care. Richard D. Klausner, director of the National Cancer Institute, laments that U.S. government funding for the fight against cancer, which in 1996 was about $2 billion, has barely kept up with inflation over the past 10 years. Such belt-tightening means, as Donald S. Coffey of the Johns Hopkins University School of Medicine wrote in an editorial for the journal Cancer, that there are "hundreds of good leads that cannot be followed today because of limited funds." He also asserts that the federal government has never mounted a war against cancer at all: "Total federal research funding per year for the two leading cancers diagnosed in the U.S. male (prostate and lung) would not represent enough money to purchase three new fighter planes."

Scientists warn that the trend toward managed care, with its emphasis on cost containment, further saps progress. Insurers are increasingly reluctant to underwrite the costs of care given in clinical trials, which are the only way to test whether a new idea has any value.

For most members of society, however, the consuming issues are not statistical and political but personal and medical. What are the latest findings about how cancer develops and becomes lethal? What is the most up-to-date thinking on how to prevent, detect and treat cancer? Which findings are most likely to extend and save lives? Those answers can be found in these pages.

Together the following chapters suggest that within the foreseeable future physicians will be able to determine from just a drop of blood or urine whether a person is at special risk for a cancer or has an unnoticed microscopic tumor. For people at risk, various prevention strategies—from changes in behavior to prophylactic medications—

may be available. For those who already have cancer, analysis of the tumor's genes will reveal how aggressive it is, whether it needs extensive treatment, and which therapies might be effective. By tailoring prevention and treatment approaches to fit these profiles, doctors will finally succeed in making cancer much less deadly and frightening. "These are milestones we can achieve, not promises we cannot keep," Klausner insists.

Some researchers striving for these goals are beginning to view cancer as a disease that might be managed over the long term, even when it cannot be cured. Eradicating every ominous cell from a cancer patient's body is a difficult goal—and in many cases, it may not be possible or necessary. After all, millions of people prosper despite chronic conditions such as diabetes and asthma. If physicians can help currently untreatable patients enjoy a more fulfilling span of pain-free years, that should count as a meaningful achievement. The day of complete cancer management may not yet be here, but the tools that medicine has now are a start.

Of course, the ultimate goal remains unchanged. As Robert A. Weinberg of the Whitehead Institute observes, "We have to keep our eye on the prize—which is to kill the tumor." Medical research should never give up on that quest for a cancer cure. Still, in the interim, it is heartening to know that in this war on cancer, even if total victory is not at hand, we might still add good years of life through strategies of containment.

# FUNDAMENTAL UNDERSTANDINGS

Cancer begins when a cell breaks free from the normal restraints on uncontrolled growth and spread. Recent progress in understanding the dangerous changes in cell behavior has been extraordinary. These findings are the basis for many of today's most exciting ideas for improving care.

# How Cancer Arises

*An explosion of research is uncovering the long-hidden molecular underpinnings of cancer—and suggesting new therapies.*

• • •

Robert A. Weinberg

How cancer develops is no longer a mystery. During the past two decades, investigators have made astonishing progress in identifying the deepest bases of the process—those at the molecular level. These discoveries are robust: they will survive the scrutiny of future generations of researchers, and they will form the foundation for revolutionary approaches to treatment. No one can predict exactly when therapies targeted to the molecular alterations in cancer cells will find wide use, given that the translation of new understanding into clinical practice is complicated, slow and expensive. But the effort is now under way.

In truth, the term "cancer" refers to more than 100 forms of the disease. Almost every tissue in the body can spawn malignancies; some even yield several types. What is more, each cancer has unique features. Still, the basic processes that produce these diverse tumors appear to be quite similar. For that reason, in this chapter "cancer" is referred to in generic terms, drawing on one or another type to illustrate the rules that seem to apply universally.

The 30 trillion cells of the normal, healthy body live in a complex, interdependent condominium, regulating one another's proliferation. Indeed, normal cells reproduce only when instructed to do so by other cells in their vicinity. Such unceasing collaboration ensures that each tissue maintains a size and architecture appropriate to the body's needs.

Cancer cells, in stark contrast, violate this scheme; they become deaf to the usual controls on proliferation and follow their own internal agenda for reproduction. They also possess an even more insidious property—the ability to migrate from the site where they began, invading nearby tissues and forming masses at distant sites in the body. Tumors composed of such malignant cells become more and more aggressive over time, and they become lethal when they disrupt the tissues and organs needed for the survival of the organism as a whole.

This much is not new. But over the past 20 years, scientists have uncovered a set of basic principles that govern the development of cancer. We now know that the cells in a tumor descend from a common ancestral cell that at one point—usually decades before a tumor becomes palpable—initiated a program of inappropriate reproduction. Further, the malignant transformation of a cell comes about through the accumulation of mutations in specific classes of the genes within it. These genes provide the key to understanding the processes at the root of human cancer.

Genes are carried in the DNA molecules of the chromosomes in the cell nucleus. A gene specifies a sequence of amino acids that must be linked together to make a particular protein; the protein then carries out the work of the gene. When a gene is switched on, the cell responds by synthesizing the encoded protein. Mutations in a gene can perturb a cell by changing the amounts or the activities of the protein product.

Two gene classes, which together constitute only a small proportion of the full genetic set, play major roles in triggering cancer. In their normal configuration, they choreograph the life cycle of the cell—the intricate sequence of events by which a cell enlarges and divides. Proto-oncogenes encourage such growth, whereas tumor suppressor genes inhibit it. Collectively these two gene classes account for much of the uncontrolled cell proliferation seen in human cancers.

When mutated, proto-oncogenes can become carcinogenic oncogenes that drive excessive multiplication. The mutations may cause the proto-oncogene to yield too much of its encoded growth-stimulatory protein or an overly active form of it. Tumor suppressor genes, in contrast, contribute to cancer when they are inactivated by mutations. The resulting loss of functional suppressor proteins deprives the cell of crucial brakes that prevent inappropriate growth.

For a cancerous tumor to develop, mutations must occur in half a dozen or more of the founding cell's growth-controlling genes. Altered forms of yet other classes of genes may also participate in the creation of a malignancy, by specifically enabling a proliferating cell to become invasive or capable of spreading (metastasizing) throughout the body (see Figure 1.1).

## Signaling Systems Go Awry

Vital clues to how mutated proto-oncogenes and tumor suppressor genes contribute to cancer came from studying the roles played within the cell by the normal counterparts of these genes. After almost two decades of research, we now view the normal genetic functions with unprecedented clarity and detail.

Many proto-oncogenes code for proteins in molecular "bucket brigades" that relay growth-stimulating signals from outside the cell deep into its interior. The growth of a cell becomes deregulated when a mutation in one of its proto-oncogenes energizes a critical growth-stimulatory pathway, keeping it continuously active when it should be silent (see Figure 1.2).

These pathways within a cell receive and process growth-stimulatory signals transmitted by other cells in a tissue. Such cell-to-cell signaling usually begins when one cell secretes growth factors. After release, these proteins move through the spaces between cells and bind to specific receptors—antennalike molecules—on the surface of other cells nearby. Receptors span the outer membrane of the target cells, so that one end protrudes into the extracellular space, and the other end projects into the cell's interior, its cytoplasm. When a growth-stimulatory factor attaches to a receptor, the receptor conveys a proliferative signal to proteins in the cytoplasm. These downstream proteins then emit stimulatory signals to a succession of other proteins, in a chain that ends in the heart of the cell, its nucleus. Within the nucleus, proteins known as transcription factors respond by activating a cohort of genes that help to usher the cell through its growth cycle.

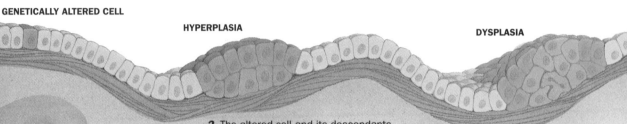

**GENETICALLY ALTERED CELL**

**HYPERPLASIA**

**DYSPLASIA**

**1** Tumor development begins when some cell (*orange*) within a normal population (*beige*) sustains a genetic mutation that increases its propensity to proliferate when it would normally rest.

**2** The altered cell and its descendants continue to look normal, but they reproduce too much—a condition termed hyperplasia. After years, one in a million of these cells (*pink*) suffers another mutation that further loosens controls on cell growth.

**3** In addition to proliferating excessively, the offspring of this cell appear abnormal in shape and in orientation; the tissue is now said to exhibit dysplasia. Once again, after a time, a rare mutation that alters cell behavior occurs (*purple*).

Some oncogenes force cells to overproduce growth factors. Sarcomas and gliomas (cancers, respectively, of connective tissues and nonneuronal brain cells) release excessive amounts of platelet-derived growth factor. A number of other cancer types secrete too much transforming growth factor alpha. These factors act, as usual, on nearby cells, but, more important, they may also turn back and drive proliferation of the same cells that just produced them.

Researchers have also identified oncogenic versions of receptor genes. The aberrant receptors specified by these oncogenes release a flood of proliferative signals into the cell cytoplasm even when no growth factors are present to urge the cell to replicate. For instance, breast cancer cells often display Erb-B2 receptor molecules that behave in this way.

Still other oncogenes in human tumors perturb parts of the signal cascade found in the cytoplasm. The best understood example comes from the *ras* family of oncogenes. The proteins encoded by normal *ras* genes transmit stimulatory signals from growth factor receptors to other proteins farther down the line. The proteins encoded by mutant *ras* genes, however, fire continuously, even when growth

factor receptors are not prompting them. Hyperactive Ras proteins are found in about a quarter of all human tumors, including carcinomas of the colon, pancreas and lung. (Carcinomas are by far the most common forms of cancer; they originate in epithelial cells, which line the body cavities and form the outer layer of the skin.)

Yet other oncogenes, such as those in the *myc* family, alter the activity of transcription factors in the nucleus. Cells normally manufacture Myc transcription factors only after they have been stimulated by growth factors impinging on the cell surface. Once made, Myc proteins activate genes that force cell growth forward. But in many types of cancer, especially malignancies of the blood-forming tissues, Myc levels are kept constantly high even in the absence of growth factors.

**Figure 1.1  TUMOR DEVELOPMENT occurs in stages. The creation of a malignant tumor in epithelial tissue is depicted schematically. Epithelial cancers are the most common malignancies and are called carcinomas. The mass seen here emerges as a result of mutations in four genes, but the number of genes involved in real tumors can vary.**

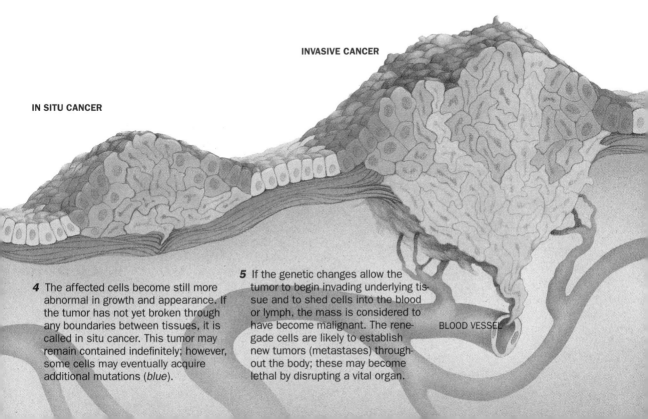

INVASIVE CANCER

IN SITU CANCER

BLOOD VESSEL

**4** The affected cells become still more abnormal in growth and appearance. If the tumor has not yet broken through any boundaries between tissues, it is called in situ cancer. This tumor may remain contained indefinitely; however, some cells may eventually acquire additional mutations (*blue*).

**5** If the genetic changes allow the tumor to begin invading underlying tissue and to shed cells into the blood or lymph, the mass is considered to have become malignant. The renegade cells are likely to establish new tumors (metastases) throughout the body; these may become lethal by disrupting a vital organ.

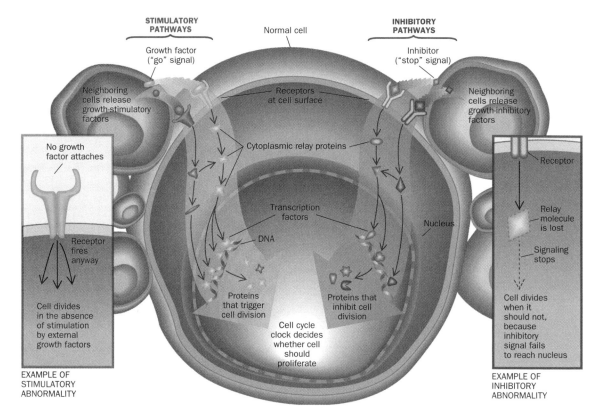

**Figure 1.2 SIGNALING PATHWAYS** in normal cells convey growth-controlling messages from the outer surface deep into the nucleus. There a molecular apparatus known as the cell cycle clock collects the messages and decides whether the cell should divide. Cancer cells often proliferate excessively because genetic mutations cause stimulatory pathways (*green*) to issue too many "go" signals or because inhibitory pathways (*red*) can no longer convey "stop" signals. A stimulatory pathway will become hyperactive if a mutation causes any component, such as a growth factor receptor (*box at left*), to issue stimulatory messages autonomously, without waiting for commands from upstream. Conversely, inhibitory pathways will shut down when some constituent, such as a cytoplasmic relay (*box at right*), is eliminated and thus breaks the signaling chain.

Discovery of trunk lines that carry proliferative messages from the cell surface to its nucleus has been more than intellectually satisfying. Because these pathways energize the multiplication of malignant cells, they constitute attractive targets for scientists intent on developing new types of anticancer therapeutics. In an exciting turn of events, as many as half a dozen pharmaceutical companies are working on drugs designed to shut down aberrantly firing growth factor receptors. At least three other companies are attempting to develop compounds that block the synthesis of aberrant Ras proteins. Both groups of agents halt excessive signaling in cultured cancer cells, but their utility in blocking the growth of tumors in animals and humans remains to be demonstrated.

## Tumor Suppressors Stop Working

To become malignant, cells must do more than overstimulate their growth-promoting machinery. They must also devise ways to evade or ignore braking signals issued by their normal neighbors in the tissue. Inhibitory messages received by a normal cell flow to the nucleus much as stimulatory signals do—via molecular bucket brigades. In cancer cells, these inhibitory brigades may be disrupted, thereby enabling the cell to ignore normally potent inhibitory signals at the surface. Critical components of these brigades, which are specified by tumor suppressor genes, are absent or inactive in many types of cancer cells.

A secreted substance called transforming growth factor beta (TGF-ß) can stop the growth of various kinds of normal cells. Some colon cancer cells become oblivious to TGF-ß by inactivating a gene that encodes a surface receptor for this substance. Some pancreatic cancers inactivate the *DPC4* gene, whose protein product may operate downstream of the growth factor receptor. And a variety of cancers discard the *p15* gene, which codes for a protein that, in response to signals from TGF-ß, normally shuts down the machinery that guides the cell through its growth cycle.

Tumor suppressor proteins can also restrain cell proliferation in other ways. Some, for example, block the flow of signals through growth-stimulatory circuits. One such suppressor is the product of the *NF-1* gene. This cytoplasmic molecule ambushes the Ras protein before it can emit its growth-promoting directives. Cells lacking *NF-1*, then, are missing an important counterbalance to Ras and to unchecked proliferation.

Various studies have shown that the introduction of a tumor suppressor gene into cancer cells that lack it can restore a degree of normalcy to the cells. This response suggests a tantalizing way of combating cancer—by providing cancer cells with intact versions of tumor suppressor genes they lost during tumor development. Although the concept is attractive, this strategy is held back by the technical difficulties still encumbering gene therapy for many diseases. Current procedures fail to deliver genes to a large proportion of the cells in a tumor. Until this logistical obstacle is surmounted, the use of gene therapy to cure cancer will remain a highly appealing but unfulfilled idea.

## The Clock Is Struck

Over the past five years, impressive evidence has uncovered the destination of stimulatory and inhibitory pathways in the cell. They converge on a molecular apparatus in the cell nucleus that is often referred to as the cell cycle clock (see Figure 1.3). The clock is the executive decision maker of the cell, and it apparently runs amok in virtually all types of human cancer. In the normal cell, the clock integrates the mixture of growth-regulating signals received by the cell and decides whether the cell should pass through its life cycle. If the answer is positive, the clock leads the process.

The cell cycle is composed of four stages. In the $G_1$ (gap 1) phase, the cell increases in size and pre-pares to copy its DNA. This copying occurs in the next stage, termed S (for synthesis), and enables the cell to duplicate precisely its complement of chromosomes. After the chromosomes are replicated, a second gap period, termed $G_2$, follows during which the cell prepares itself for M (mitosis)—the time when the enlarged parent cell finally divides in half to produce its two daughters, each of which is endowed with a complete set of chromosomes. The new daughter cells immediately enter $G_1$ and may go through the full cycle again. Alternatively, they may stop cycling temporarily or permanently.

The cell cycle clock programs this elaborate succession of events by means of a variety of molecules. Its two essential components, cyclins and cyclin-dependent kinases (CDKs), associate with one another and initiate entrance into the various stages of the cell cycle. In $G_1$, for instance, D-type cyclins bind to CDKs 4 or 6, and the resulting complexes act on a powerful growth-inhibitory molecule—the protein known as pRB. This action releases the braking effect of pRB and enables the cell to progress into late $G_1$ and thence into S (DNA synthesis) phase (see *b* in Figure 1.3).

Various inhibitory proteins can restrain forward movement through the cycle. Among them are p15 (mentioned earlier) and p16, both of which block the activity of the CDK partners of cyclin D, thus preventing the advance of the cell from $G_1$ into S. Another inhibitor of CDKs, termed p21, can act throughout the cell cycle. P21 is under control of a tumor suppressor protein, p53, that monitors the health of the cell, the integrity of its chromosomal DNA and the successful completion of the different steps in the cycle.

Breast cancer cells often produce excesses of cyclin D and cyclin E. In many cases of melanoma, skin cells have lost the gene encoding the braking protein p16. Half of all types of human tumors lack a functional p53 protein. And in cervical cancers (see Figure 1.4) triggered by infection of cells with a human papillomavirus, both the pRB and p53 proteins are frequently disabled, eliminating two of the clock's most vital restraints. The end result in all these cases is that the clock begins to spin out of control, ignoring any external warnings to stop. If investigators can devise ways to impose clamps on the cyclins and CDKs active in the cell cycle, they may be able to halt cancer cells in their tracks.

I have so far discussed two ways that our tissues normally hold down cell proliferation and avoid

## *a*

**STAGES OF THE CELL CYCLE**

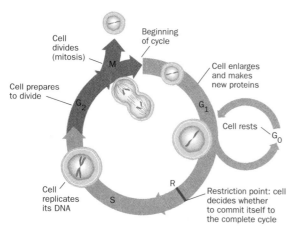

Beginning of cycle

Cell divides (mitosis)

Cell enlarges and makes new proteins

Cell prepares to divide

M

G₂

G₁

Cell rests

G₀

Cell replicates its DNA

S

R

Restriction point: cell decides whether to commit itself to the complete cycle

## *b*

**A MOLECULAR "SWITCH"**

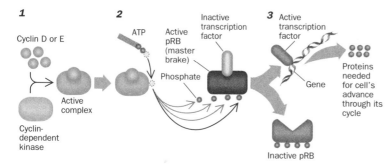

**1**

Cyclin D or E

Cyclin-dependent kinase

Active complex

**2**

ATP

Active pRB (master brake)

Phosphate

Inactive transcription factor

**3** Active transcription factor

Gene

Proteins needed for cell's advance through its cycle

Inactive pRB

## *c*

**THE CELL CYCLE CLOCK IN ACTION**

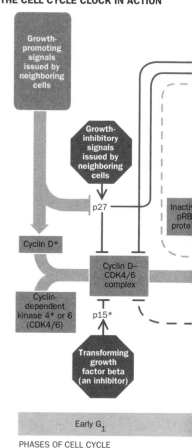

Growth-promoting signals issued by neighboring cells

Growth-inhibitory signals issued by neighboring cells

p27

Inactiv pRB prote

Cyclin D*

Cyclin D–CDK4/6 complex

Cyclin-dependent kinase 4* or 6 (CDK4/6)

p15*

Transforming growth factor beta (an inhibitor)

Early G₁

PHASES OF CELL CYCLE

**Figure 1.3 THE CELL CYCLE CLOCK and cancer.** The cell cycle clock—composed of an assembly of interacting proteins in the nucleus—normally integrates messages from the stimulatory and inhibitory pathways and, if the stimulatory messages win out, programs a cell's advance through its cycle of growth and division. Progression through the four stages of the cell cycle (*a*) is driven by rising levels of proteins called cyclins: the D type, followed by E, A and B.

A crucial step in the cycle occurs late in G₁ at the restriction point (R), when the cell decides whether to commit itself to completing the cycle. For the cell to pass R and enter S, a molecular "switch" (*b*) must be flipped from "off" to "on." As levels of cyclin D cyclin E rise, these proteins combine with and activate cyclin-dependent kinases (1). The kinases grab phosphate groups (2) from molecules of ATP (adenosine triphosphate) and transfer them to the

cancer. They prevent excess multiplication by depriving a cell of growth-stimulatory factors or, conversely, by showering it with antiproliferative factors. Still, as we have seen, cells on their way to becoming cancerous often circumvent these controls: they stimulate themselves and turn a deaf ear

to inhibitory signals. Prepared for such eventualities, the human body equips cells with certain backup systems that guard against runaway division. But additional mutations in the cell's genetic repertoire can overcome even these defenses and contribute to cancer.

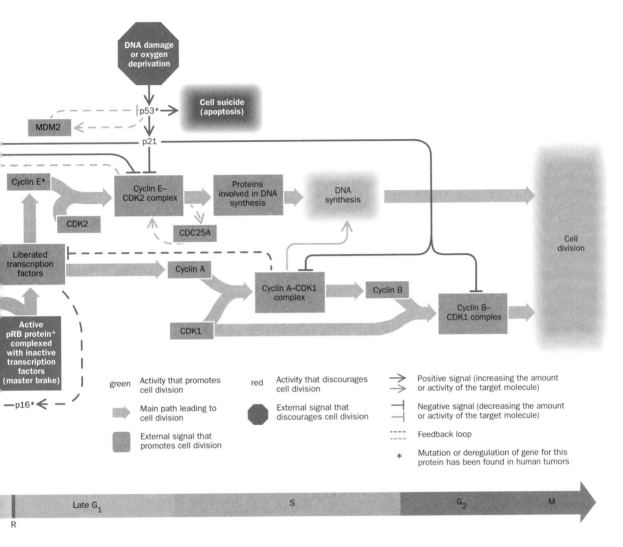

protein pRB, the master brake. When pRB lacks phosphates, it actively blocks cycling (and keeps the switch in the "off" position) by sequestering other proteins termed transcription factors. But after the cyclin-kinase complexes add enough phosphates to pRB, the brake stops working (3); it releases the factors, freeing them to act on genes. The liberated factors then spur production of various proteins required for progression through the cell cycle. In c, the switch is placed in the larger context of the many molecular interactions that regulate the cell cycle. Flipping the switch to "on" can be seen above the R point. Overactivity of the stimulatory proteins cyclin D, cyclin E and CDK4 have been implicated in certain human cancers. Inactivation of various inhibitory proteins has also been documented. The affected proteins include p53, pRB, p16 and p15.

## Fail-Safe Systems Fail

One such backup system, present in each human cell, provokes the cell to commit suicide (undergo "apoptosis") if some of its essential components are damaged or if its control systems are deregulated. For example, injury to chromosomal DNA can trigger apoptosis. Further, recent work from a number of laboratories indicates that creation of an oncogene or the disabling of a tumor suppressor gene within a cell can also induce this response. Destruction of a damaged cell is bad for the cell itself but makes sense for the body as a whole: the potential dangers posed to the organism by carcinogenic mutations are far greater than the small price paid in the loss of a single cell. The tumors that emerge in our tissues, then, would seem to arise from the rare, genetically disturbed cell that somehow succeeds in evading the apoptotic program hardwired into its control circuitry.

Developing cancer cells devise several means of evading apoptosis. The p53 protein, among its many functions, helps to trigger cell suicide; its inactivation by many tumor cells reduces the likelihood that genetically troubled cells will be eliminated. Cancer cells may also make excessive amounts of the protein Bcl-2, which wards off apoptosis efficiently.

Recently scientists have realized that this ability to escape apoptosis may endanger patients not only by contributing to the expansion of a tumor but also by making the resulting tumors resistant to therapy. For years, it was assumed that radiation therapy and many chemotherapeutic drugs killed malignant cells directly, by wreaking widespread havoc in their DNA. We now know that the treatments often harm DNA to a relatively minor extent. Nevertheless, the affected cells perceive that the inflicted damage cannot be repaired easily, and they actively kill themselves. This discovery implies that cancer cells able to evade apoptosis will be far less responsive to treatment. By the same token, it suggests that therapies able to restore a cell's capacity for suicide could combat cancer by improving the effectiveness of existing radiation and chemotherapeutic treatment strategies.

A second defense against runaway proliferation, quite distinct from the apoptotic program, is built into our cells as well. This mechanism counts and limits the total number of times cells can reproduce themselves.

## Cells Become Immortal

Much of what is known about this safeguard has been learned from studies of cells cultured in a petri dish. When cells are taken from a mouse or human embryo and grown in culture, the population doubles every day or so. But after a predictable number of doublings—50 to 60 in human cells—growth stops, at which point the cells are said to be senescent. That, at least, is what happens when cells have intact *RB* and *p53* genes. Cells that sustain inactivating mutations in either of these genes continue to divide after their normal counterparts enter senescence. Eventually, though, the survivors reach a second stage, termed crisis, in which they die in large numbers. An occasional cell in this dying population, however, will escape crisis and become immortal: it and its descendants will multiply indefinitely.

These events imply the existence of a mechanism that counts the number of doublings through which a cell population has passed. During the past several years, scientists have discovered the molecular device that does this counting. DNA segments at the ends of chromosomes, known as telomeres, tally the number of replicative generations through which cell populations pass and, at appropriate times, initiate senescence and crisis. In so doing, they circumscribe the ability of cell populations to expand indefinitely [see "Telomeres, Telomerase and Cancer," by Carol W. Greider and Elizabeth H. Blackburn; SCIENTIFIC AMERICAN, February 1996].

Like the plastic tips on shoelaces, the telomere caps protect chromosomal ends from damage. In

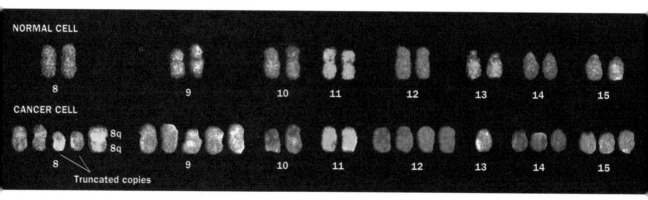

NORMAL CELL

8    9    10    11    12    13    14    15

CANCER CELL

8q
8q

8    9    10    11    12    13    14    15

Truncated copies

most human cells, telomeres shorten a bit every time chromosomes are replicated during the S phase of the cell cycle. Once the telomeres shrink below some threshold length, they sound an alarm that instructs cells to enter senescence. If cells bypass senescence, further shrinkage of the telomere will eventually trigger crisis: extreme shortening of the telomeres will cause the chromosomes in a cell to fuse with one another or to break apart, creating genetic chaos that is fatal to the cell.

If the telomere-based counting system operated properly in cancerous cells, their excessive proliferation would be aborted long before tumors became very large. Dangerous expansion would be stemmed by the senescence program or, if the cell evaded that blockade, by disruption of the chromosomal array at crisis. But this last defense is breached during the development of most cancer cells, overcome by activation of a gene that codes for the enzyme telomerase.

This enzyme, virtually absent from most healthy cell types but present in almost all tumor cells, systematically replaces telomeric segments that are usually trimmed away during each cell cycle. In so doing, it maintains the integrity of the telomeres and thereby enables cells to replicate endlessly. The resulting cell immortality can be troublesome in a couple of ways. Obviously, it allows tumors to grow large. It also gives precancerous or already cancerous cells time to accumulate additional mutations that will increase their ability to replicate, invade and ultimately metastasize.

From the point of view of a cancer cell, production of a single enzyme is a clever way to topple the mortality barrier. Yet dependence on one enzyme may represent an Achilles' heel as well. If telom-erase could be blocked in cancer cells, their telomeres would once again shrink whenever they divided, pushing these cells into crisis and death. For that reason, a number of pharmaceutical firms are attempting to develop drugs that target telomerase.

## Why Some Cancers Appear Early

It normally takes decades for an incipient tumor to collect all the mutations required for its malignant growth. In some individuals, however, the time for tumor development is clearly compressed; they contract certain types of cancer decades before the typical age of onset of these cancers. How can tumor formation be accelerated?

In many cases, this early onset is explained by the inheritance from one or the other parent of a mutant cancer-causing gene. As a fertilized egg begins to divide and replicate, the set of genes provided by the sperm and egg is copied and distributed to all the body's cells. Now a typically rare event—a mutation in a critical growth-controlling gene—becomes ubiquitous, because the mutation is implanted in all the body's cells, not merely in some randomly stricken cell. In other words, the process of tumor formation leapfrogs over one of its early, slowly occurring steps, accelerating the process as a whole. As a consequence, tumor development, which usually requires three or four decades to reach completion, may culminate in one or two. Because such mutant genes can pass from generation to generation, many members of a family may be at risk for the early development of cancer.

An inherited form of colon cancer provides a dramatic example. Most cases of colon cancer occur

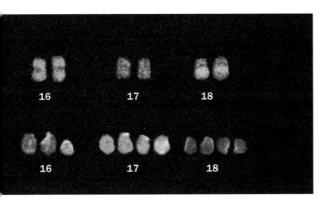

Figure 1.4 HUMAN CHROMOSOMES from a normal dividing cell (*top*) occur as identical pairs; those numbered 8 to 18 are shown. Chromosomes from a cervical cancer cell (*bottom*), in contrast, display many abnormalities. Chromosome 8, for instance, exhibits three disturbances: gain of copy number; deletion of genetic material from individual copies; and breakage followed by joining of segments that do not belong together (*far right in 8*). Copy loss, as in chromosome 13, is also common. These various changes can favor tumor progression if they activate an oncogene, increase the copies of an oncogene or eliminate a tumor suppressor gene. The images were generated by spectral karyotyping, a new method for analyzing chromosomes.

# Some Genes Involved in Human Cancers

Genes known as proto-oncogenes code for proteins that stimulate cell division; mutated forms, called oncogenes, can cause the stimulatory proteins to be overactive, with the result that cells proliferate excessively. Tumor suppressor genes code for proteins that inhibit cell division. Mutations can cause the proteins to be inactivated and may thus deprive cells of needed restraints on proliferation. Investigators are still trying to decipher the specific functions of many tumor suppressor genes.

## ONCOGENES

*Genes for growth factors or their receptors*

| | |
|---|---|
| PDGF | Codes for platelet-derived growth factor. Involved in glioma (a brain cancer) |
| erb-B | Codes for the receptor for epidermal growth factor. Involved in glioblastoma (a brain cancer) and breast cancer |
| erb-B2 | Also called *HER-2* or *neu*. Codes for a growth factor receptor. Involved in breast, salivary gland and ovarian cancers |
| RET | Codes for a growth factor receptor. Involved in thyroid cancer |

*Genes for cytoplasmic relays in stimulatory signaling pathways*

| | |
|---|---|
| Ki-ras | Involved in lung, ovarian, colon and pancreatic cancers |
| N-ras | Involved in leukemias |

*Genes for transcription factors that activate growth-promoting genes*

| | |
|---|---|
| c-myc | Involved in leukemias and breast, stomach and lung cancers |
| N-myc | Involved in neuroblastoma (a nerve cell cancer) and glioblastoma |
| L-myc | Involved in lung cancer |

*Genes for other kinds of molecules*

| | |
|---|---|
| Bcl-2 | Codes for a protein that normally blocks cell suicide. Involved in follicular B cell lymphoma |
| Bcl-1 | Also called *PRAD1*. Codes for cyclin D1, a stimulatory component of the cell cycle clock. Involved in breast, head and neck cancers |
| MDM2 | Codes for an antagonist of the p53 tumor suppressor protein. Involved in sarcomas (connective tissue cancers) and other cancers |

## TUMOR SUPPRESSOR GENES

*Genes for proteins in the cytoplasm*

| | |
|---|---|
| APC | Involved in colon and stomach cancers |
| DPC4 | Codes for a relay molecule in a signaling pathway that inhibits cell division. Involved in pancreatic cancer |
| NF-1 | Codes for a protein that inhibits a stimulatory (Ras) protein. Involved in neurofibroma and pheochromocytoma (cancers of the peripheral nervous system) and myeloid leukemia |
| NF-2 | Involved in meningioma and ependymoma (brain cancers) and schwannoma (affecting the wrapping around peripheral nerves) |

*Genes for proteins in the nucleus*

| | |
|---|---|
| MTS1 | Codes for the p16 protein, a braking component of the cell cycle clock. Involved in a wide range of cancers |
| RB | Codes for the pRB protein, a master brake of the cell cycle. Involved in retinoblastoma and bone, bladder, small cell lung and breast cancer |
| p53 | Codes for the p53 protein, which can halt cell division and induce abnormal cells to kill themselves. Involved in a wide range of cancers |
| WT1 | Involved in Wilms' tumor of the kidney |

*Genes for proteins whose cellular location is not yet clear*

| | |
|---|---|
| BRCA1 | Involved in breast and ovarian cancers |
| BRCA2 | Involved in breast cancer |
| VHL | Involved in renal cell cancer |

sporadically, the results of random genetic events occurring during a person's lifetime. In certain families, however, many individuals are afflicted with early-onset colonic tumors, preordained by an inherited gene. In the sporadic cases, a rare mutation silences a tumor suppressor gene called *APC* in an intestinal epithelial cell. The resulting proliferation of the mutant cell yields a benign polyp that may eventually progress to a malignant carcinoma. But defective forms of *APC* may pass from parents to children in certain families. Members of these families develop hundreds, even thousands of colonic polyps during the first decades of life, some of which are likely to become transformed into carcinomas.

The list of familial cancer syndromes that are now traceable directly to inheritance of mutant tumor suppressor genes is growing. For instance, inherited defective versions of the gene for *pRB* often lead to development of an eye cancer—retinoblastoma—in children; later in life the mutations account for a greatly increased risk of osteosarcomas (bone cancers). Mutant inherited versions of the *p53* tumor suppressor gene yield tumors at multiple sites, a condition known as the Li-Fraumeni syndrome (named in part for Frederick Li, co-author of Chapter 3, "What Causes Cancer?"). And the recently isolated *BRCA1* and *BRCA2* genes seem to account for the bulk of familial breast cancers, encompassing as many as 20 percent of all premenopausal breast cancers in this country and a substantial proportion of familial ovarian cancers as well.

Early onset of tumors is sometimes explained by inheritance of mutations in another class of genes as well. As I implied earlier, most people avoid cancer until late in life or indefinitely because they enter the world with pristine genes. During the course of a lifetime, however, our genes are attacked by carcinogens imported into our bodies from the environment and also by chemicals produced in our own cells. And genetic errors may be introduced when the enzymes that replicate DNA during cell cycling make copying mistakes. For the most part, such errors are rapidly corrected by a repair system that operates in every cell. Should the repair system slip up and fail to erase an error, the damage will become a permanent mutation in one of the cell's genes and in that same gene in all descendant cells.

The system's high repair efficiency is one reason many decades can pass before all the mutations needed for a malignancy to develop will, by chance, come together within a single cell. Certain inherited defects, though, can accelerate tumor development through a particularly insidious means: they impair the operation of proteins that repair damaged DNA. As a result, mutations that would normally accumulate slowly will appear with alarming frequency throughout the DNA of cells. Among the affected genes are inevitably those controlling cell proliferation.

Such is the case in another inherited colon cancer, hereditary nonpolyposis colon cancer. Afflicted individuals make defective versions of a protein responsible for repairing the copying mistakes made by the DNA replication apparatus. Because of this impairment, colonic cells cannot fix DNA damage efficiently; they therefore collect mutations rapidly, accelerating cancer development by two decades or more. People affected by another familial cancer syndrome, xeroderma pigmentosum, have inherited a defective copy of a gene that directs the repair of DNA damaged by ultraviolet rays. These patients are prone to several types of sunlight-induced skin cancer.

Similarly, cells of people born with a defective *ATM* gene have difficulty recognizing the presence of certain lesions in the DNA and mobilizing the appropriate repair response. These people are susceptible to neurological degeneration, blood vessel malformation and a variety of tumors. Some researchers have proposed that as many as 10 percent of inherited breast cancers may arise in patients with a defective copy of this gene.

Over the next decade, the list of cancer susceptibility genes will grow dramatically, one of the fruits of the Human Genome Project (which seeks to identify every gene in the human cell). Together with the increasingly powerful tools of DNA analysis, knowledge of these genes will enable us to predict which members of cancer-prone families are at high risk and which have, through good fortune, inherited intact copies of these genes.

## Beyond Proliferation

Although we have learned an enormous amount about the genetic basis of runaway cell proliferation, we still know rather little about the mutant genes that contribute to later stages of tumor development, specifically those that allow tumor cells to attract blood vessels for nourishment, to invade nearby tissues and to metastasize. But research in these areas is moving rapidly. (Judah Folkman describes the ingenuity of tumor cells in generating their own blood supply in Chapter 11, "Fighting Cancer by Attacking Its Blood Supply." Erkki Ruoslahti takes up metastasis in Chapter 2, "How Cancer Spreads.")

We are within striking distance of writing the detailed life histories of many human tumors from start to life-threatening finish. These biographies will be written in the language of genes and molecules. Within a decade, we will know with extraordinary precision the succession of events that constitute the complex evolution of normal cells into highly malignant, invasive derivatives.

By then, we may come to understand why certain localized masses never progress beyond their benign, noninvasive form to confront us with aggressive malignancy. Such benign growths can be found in almost every organ of the body. Perhaps we will also discern why certain mutant genes contribute to the formation of some types of cancer but not others. For example, mutant versions of the RB tumor suppressor gene appear often in retinoblastoma, bladder carcinoma and small cell lung carcinoma but are seen only occasionally in breast and colon carcinomas. Very likely, many of the solutions to these mysteries will flow from research in developmental biology (embryology). After all, the genes that govern embryonic development are, much later, the sources of our malignancies.

By any measure, the amount of information gathered over the past two decades about the origins of cancer is without parallel in the history of biomedical research. Some of this knowledge has already been put to good use, to build molecular tools for detecting and determining the aggressiveness of certain types of cancer, as David Sidransky discusses in Chapter 6, "Advances in Cancer Detection." Still, despite so much insight into cause, new curative therapies have so far remained elusive. One reason is that tumor cells differ only minimally from healthy ones; a minute fraction of the tens of thousands of genes in a cell suffers damage during malignant transformation. Thus, normal friend and malignant foe are woven of very similar cloth, and any fire directed against the enemy may do as much damage to normal tissue as to the intended target.

Yet the course of the battle is changing. The differences between normal and cancer cells may be subtle, but they are real. And the unique characteristics of tumors provide excellent targets for intervention by newly developed drugs (see Part V, "Therapies of the Future"). The development of targeted anticancer therapeutics is still in its infancy. This enterprise will soon move from hit-or-miss, serendipitous discovery to rational design and accurate targeting. I suspect that the first decade of the new century will reward us with cancer therapies that earlier generations could not have dreamed possible. Then this nation's long investment in basic cancer research will begin to pay off handsomely.

# How Cancer Spreads

*Tumor cells roam the body by evading the controls that
keep normal cells in place. That fact offers clues to fighting cancer.*

. . .

Erkki Ruoslahti

Our body is a community of cells, in which each cell occupies a place appropriate for its tasks on behalf of the whole. With the exception of white blood cells, which patrol the body for microbial invaders and tissue damage, normal cells stay in the tissue of which they are part. Cancer cells, however, are rogues that trespass aggressively into other tissues.

Metastasis, the spread of cancer to distant sites in the body, is in fact what makes cancer so lethal. A surgeon can remove a primary tumor relatively easily, but a cancer that has metastasized usually reaches so many places that cure by surgery alone becomes impossible. For that reason, metastasis and the invasion of normal tissue by cancer cells are the hallmarks of malignancy (see Figure 2.1). In countries where health care is primitive, one sometimes sees people who live with tumors as big as a soccer ball; the cells that make up these so-called benign tumors obviously overproliferate, but unlike malignant cancer cells, they do not invade or metastasize.

Acquiring the capabilities needed to emigrate to another tissue is therefore a key event in the devel-

opment of a cancer. To metastasize successfully, cancer cells have to detach from their original location, invade a blood or lymphatic vessel, travel in the circulation to a distant site and establish a new cellular colony. At every one of these steps, they must escape many controls that, in effect, keep normal cells in place.

A fruitful way of understanding how tumor cells evade these controls has consequently been to study the signals that normally direct cells to their place in the body and keep them there during adulthood. When I was a postdoctoral fellow at the California Institute of Technology from 1968 to 1970, my mentor, William J. Dreyer, had become interested in those questions. Roger W. Sperry, also at Caltech, had found that the light-sensing nerve cells in the retina of the eye grow orderly extensions into the brain such that the extensions from a given retinal region always project into the same brain region. These findings inspired Dreyer and Leroy E. Hood to postulate their "area code" hypothesis, that a cell has on its surface an address system—written in one set of molecules and readable by molecules on other cells—that identifies where the cell should be.

It seemed to me at the time that if a molecular address system existed, something had to be wrong with it in cancer, because cancer cells did not stay put. I decided to try to find such molecules. As the work of many laboratories eventually showed, area code molecules do exist. They mediate cell adhesion, the anchoring of cells to adjacent structures (see Figure 2.2).

In normal tissues, cells adhere both to one another and to an insoluble meshwork of protein filling the space between them, known as extracellular matrix. (This arrangement is particularly descriptive of the epithelia, which are the cell layers that form the outer surface of the skin and the lining of the gut, lungs and some other organs, and from which most

cancer originates.) The two kinds of adhesion (see Figure 2.3) play different critical roles during tissue invasion and metastasis.

Cell-cell adhesion molecules appear to help keep cells in place; these molecules seem to be missing or compromised in cancer cells. For example, various kinds of cancers lose some or all of an intercellular adhesion molecule called E-cadherin. By manipulating this molecule in cultured cancer cells, one can change the cells' ability to invade tissues and form tumors. Walter Birchmeier, now at the Max Delbrück Center in Berlin, first showed that blocking the function of E-cadherin can turn a cultured lineage of cells from noninvasive to invasive. Conversely, restoring E-cadherin to cancer cells that lack it can negate their ability to form tumors when they are injected into mice. Thus, loosening of the

Figure 2.1 INVASION AND METASTASIS are the processes that lethally spread cancer cells throughout the body. First, cancer cells detach from the primary site (which is often in an epithelial tissue) and breach the basement membrane separating them from other tissue layers. Some of these invasive cells can penetrate the basement membrane surrounding a blood vessel, as well as the layer of endothelial cells lining it. The cells are then free to circulate via the bloodstream. Eventually a cancer cell may lodge in a capillary. If it then adheres to and penetrates the capillary wall again, it can create a secondary tumor. Perhaps fewer than one in 10,000 cancer cells that escape the primary tumor survives to colonize another tissue.

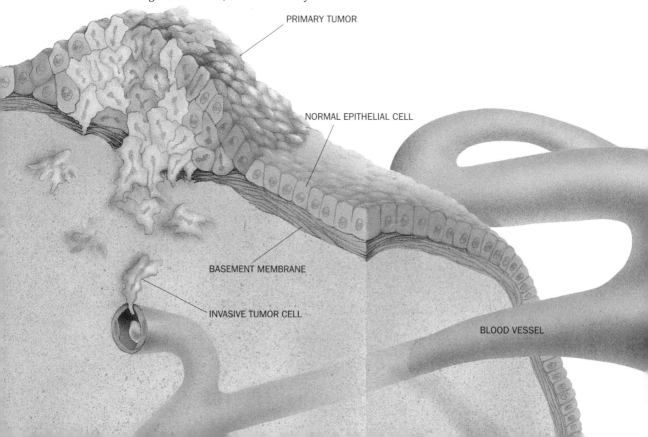

PRIMARY TUMOR

NORMAL EPITHELIAL CELL

BASEMENT MEMBRANE

INVASIVE TUMOR CELL

BLOOD VESSEL

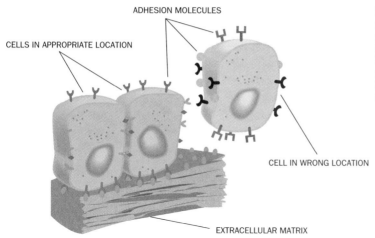

ADHESION MOLECULES

CELLS IN APPROPRIATE LOCATION

CELL IN WRONG LOCATION

EXTRACELLULAR MATRIX

Figure 2.2 "AREA CODES" FOR CELLS take the form of specific surface adhesion molecules and receptors. During development, a normal cell recognizes its proper place in the body by fitting its adhesion molecules to those on other cells and on the extracellular matrix. In cancer, something goes wrong with this address system.

adhesive restraint between cells is likely to be an important early step in cancer invasion.

## The Need for Adhesion

Adhesion to extracellular matrix, on the other hand, allows cells to survive and proliferate. As researchers have known for many years, cultured cells cannot reproduce until they attach to a surface, a phenomenon called anchorage dependence. This attachment is mediated by cell-surface molecules known as integrins that bind to the extracellular matrix. As Steven Frisch of the Burnham Institute in La Jolla, Calif., Martin A. Schwartz of the Scripps Research Institute, also in La Jolla, Calif., and Mina J. Bissell of the University of California at Berkeley have shown, only attachments involving integrins can satisfy the requirements of anchorage dependence.

My laboratory at the Burnham Institute, together with Tony Hunter of the Salk Institute for Biological Studies in San Diego, Calif., has recently shown

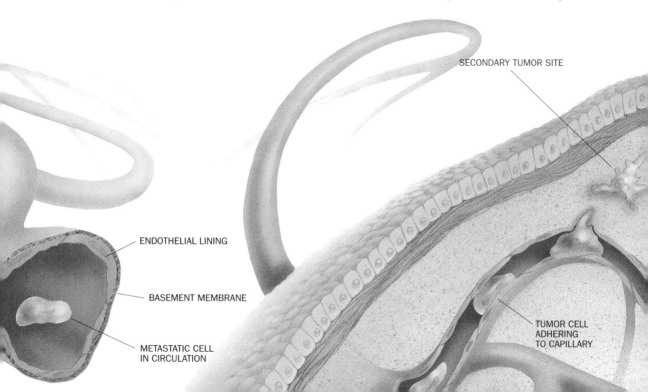

SECONDARY TUMOR SITE

ENDOTHELIAL LINING

BASEMENT MEMBRANE

METASTATIC CELL
IN CIRCULATION

TUMOR CELL
ADHERING
TO CAPILLARY

**CELLULAR ADHESION**

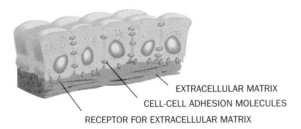

EXTRACELLULAR MATRIX
CELL-CELL ADHESION MOLECULES
RECEPTOR FOR EXTRACELLULAR MATRIX

**IMPORTANCE OF CELL-CELL ADHESION**

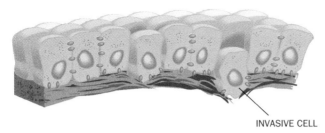

INVASIVE CELL

**IMPORTANCE OF ADHESION TO EXTRACELLULAR MATRIX**

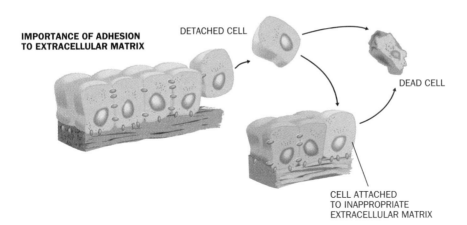

DETACHED CELL

DEAD CELL

CELL ATTACHED TO INAPPROPRIATE EXTRACELLULAR MATRIX

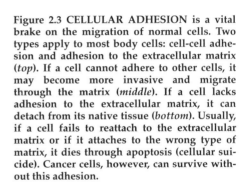

**Figure 2.3 CELLULAR ADHESION is a vital brake on the migration of normal cells. Two types apply to most body cells: cell-cell adhesion and adhesion to the extracellular matrix (*top*). If a cell cannot adhere to other cells, it may become more invasive and migrate through the matrix (*middle*). If a cell lacks adhesion to the extracellular matrix, it can detach from its native tissue (*bottom*). Usually, if a cell fails to reattach to the extracellular matrix or if it attaches to the wrong type of matrix, it dies through apoptosis (cellular suicide). Cancer cells, however, can survive without this adhesion.**

that unattached cells stop growing because one of the nuclear proteins (known as the cyclin E–CDK2 complex) that regulates the growth and division of cells becomes less active. Inhibitory substances in the nuclei of these cells seem to shut down this protein.

As Frisch, Schwartz and Bissell also discovered, when many types of cells are denied anchorage, they not only stop proliferating but commit suicide. That is, they spontaneously undergo specific changes that lead to their own death. This kind of cell death, in which the cell is an active participant, has been termed apoptosis.

My group has demonstrated that for cells to survive, the extracellular matrix to which they adhere must bear the right "area code," one that is probably found only in the extracellular matrix of select tissues. Moreover, they have to use the appropriate integrin to attach to the matrix. As all these results show, a molecular explanation for anchorage dependence is beginning to take shape, although much more critical detail still needs to be filled in.

Cellular suicide from lack of anchorage or from inappropriate anchorage is likely to be one of the safeguards that maintain the integrity of tissues. Cells usually cannot just float away from their tissue and establish themselves somewhere else, because they will die on the way. Yet cancer cells get around this requirement; they are anchorage independent. The cyclin E–CDK2 complex in such cells stays active whether the cells are attached or not.

How cancer cells accomplish this trick is not fully understood, but it seems that oncogenes can be blamed. (Oncogenes are mutated versions of normal genes called proto-oncogenes; these mutations can turn normal cells into malignant ones; see Chapter 1, "How Cancer Arises.") In effect, as various experiments have shown, proteins made by these oncogenes convey a false message to the nucleus that the cell is properly attached when it is not, thereby stopping the cell from arresting its own growth and dying through apoptosis.

Anchorage dependence is only one of the constraints that a cancer cell must overcome to roam around the body. Epithelial cells, the most common sources of cancers, are separated from the rest of the body by a basement membrane, a thin layer of specialized extracellular matrix. Basement membranes form a barrier that most normal cells cannot breach, but cancer cells can [see "Cancer Cell Invasion and Metastasis," by Lance A. Liotta; SCIENTIFIC AMERICAN, February 1992].

This fact can be strikingly demonstrated by giving cells in a test tube an opportunity to invade through a natural or reconstructed basement membrane: cancer cells will penetrate it; normal ones will not. Furthermore, in this experiment, cells from metastatic cancers generally invade faster than those from nonmetastatic tumors. White blood cells, in keeping with their role as security patrol, are an exception to the rule that normal cells do not invade—they, too, are adept at penetrating tissues, including basement membranes. Cancer cells and white blood cells do so by releasing enzymes, called metalloproteinases, that dissolve basement membranes and other extracellular matrices. Other cells have less of these enzymes and more enzyme inhibitors.

After a cancer cell has passed through the basement membrane separating it from the rest of the tissue at its original site, it soon encounters another basement membrane, one surrounding a small blood vessel. (A blood vessel is usually nearby, because to sustain themselves successful tumors induce the growth of new blood vessels.) By penetrating this second basement membrane barrier and the layer of endothelial cells that form the vessel's inner lining, the cancer cell gains access to the bloodstream and is carried elsewhere in the body.

New technology makes it possible to detect cancer cells in the blood of patients. Great strides have been made in identifying telltale marker molecules that distinguish a cell as having come from a specific tissue or type of tumor. At the same time, researchers have also developed ultrasensitive assays (based on such techniques as the polymerase chain reaction and monoclonal-antibody tagging) for detecting those molecules. From studies employing these methods, we know that malignant cells are often circulating even when a clinical examination cannot yet find evidence of the cancer's distant spread.

The further development of such tests may eventually improve therapies, by helping physicians determine whether they need to prescribe treatments beyond surgery for seemingly contained tumors. Detection of micrometastases in the blood and elsewhere in the body is a significant step forward in early diagnosis, and it is the vanguard of applied research on metastasis.

Some doctors have also wondered whether the manipulation of a tumor during its diagnosis or surgical removal might be enough to release cells into the circulation. The new testing methods should allow researchers to prove or disprove this ominous hypothesis, but to my knowledge, that has not yet been done. But even if the hypothesis proves to be correct, it is clear that the benefits of diagnostics and surgery far outweigh the possible risks from inaction.

## Vulnerable in the Blood

Fortunately, even when cancer cells do get into the circulation, the formation of secondary tumors is not inevitable. The circulating cell still faces several more hurdles: it must attach to the inner lining of a blood vessel, cross through it, penetrate the basement membrane at this new location, then invade the tissues beyond and begin multiplying. Each of these obstacles makes demands of the tumor cell that may go beyond those it faced in its home tissue. Furthermore, it may also be that many cancers cannot entirely overcome the defense mechanisms that keep our cells in the right places—another hindrance to metastasis.

Probably fewer than one in 10,000 of the cancer cells that reach the circulation survive to found a new tumor at a distant site. The reasons for this apparent vulnerability while in the blood are not

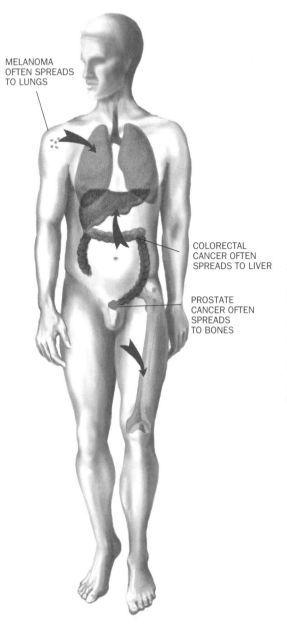

MELANOMA
OFTEN SPREADS
TO LUNGS

COLORECTAL
CANCER OFTEN
SPREADS TO LIVER

PROSTATE
CANCER OFTEN
SPREADS
TO BONES

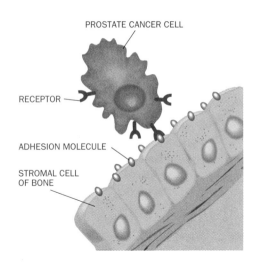

PROSTATE CANCER CELL

RECEPTOR

ADHESION MOLECULE

STROMAL CELL
OF BONE

**Figure 2.4 PATTERNS OF METASTASIS** can be explained in part by the architecture of the circulatory system. Tumors in the skin and many other tissues often colonize the lungs first because the lungs contain the first capillary bed "downstream" of most organs. In contrast, because the intestines send their blood to the liver first, the liver is often the primary site of metastasis for colorectal cancers. Yet circulation is not the only factor: prostate cancer, for example, usually metastasizes to the bones. This tendency may result from an affinity between receptors on prostate tumor cells and molecules in bone tissues (*enlargement above*).

well understood—perhaps the anchorage independence of the tumor cells is not complete, and they sometimes die through apoptosis after all. In any case, researchers believe the cells need to attach fairly promptly to the inner lining of a small blood vessel.

Blood circulation explains much about why various metastatic cancers spread preferentially to certain tissues (see Figure 2.4). Circulating tumor cells usually get trapped in the first vascular bed (or network of capillaries, the finest blood vessels) that they encounter "downstream" of their origin. The first vascular bed encountered by blood leaving most organs is in the lungs; only the intestines send their blood to the liver first. Accordingly, the lungs are the most common site of metastasis, followed by the liver.

In part, cancer cells lodge in small blood vessels because these cells tend to be large. Also, some cancers produce chemical factors that cause platelets, the tiny blood cells that initiate blood clotting, to aggregate around them. These aggregates effectively make the cancer cells even larger and stickier. (It is also noteworthy that platelets produce their own rich supply of growth factors, and these may help the cancer cells to which they bind survive in the blood. This may be why, in some experimental systems, drugs that interfere with platelet functions have anticancer effects.)

Physical trapping of cancer cells in the blood vessels at the site of metastasis is not the whole story, however. If it were, cancers would not spread so diversely through the body. Indeed, some types of cancer show a striking preference for organs other than those that receive their venous blood— witness the tendency of metastatic prostate cancer to move into the bones. Once again, the explanation seems to rest with the molecular address system on cell surfaces. A specific affinity between the adhesion molecules on cancer cells and those on the inner linings of blood vessels in the preferred tissues could explain the predilection of the cells to migrate selectively. Different concentrations of growth-promoting factors and hormones in various tissues may also play a part.

Recently, in an elegant piece of work, Ivan Stamenkovic of Harvard Medical School and his colleagues showed that he could direct the metastatic spread of tumor cells: he genetically engineered mice so that their livers displayed a target for an adhesion molecule found on certain tumor cells. As predicted, the tumor cells homed in on the liver. For these experiments, Stamenkovic borrowed receptors and targets from the molecular adhesion system used by white blood cells to leave the circulation and enter tissues. Although this system was artificial, it may be that cancers naturally mimic white blood cells in much this way—cancer cells do often manufacture certain molecules (called Le$^x$) important to the mobility of white blood cells in the body.

### Finding the Body's Area Codes

If, as seems likely, there is much to be learned by identifying the molecular addresses that white blood cells and tumors use to find particular tissues, a method of doing so that Renata Pasqualini, a postdoctoral fellow in my laboratory, and I have devised should prove helpful. We adapted a technique for isolating biologically active molecules from huge collections, or "libraries," of diverse compounds. The theory behind this approach is that if one screens a sufficiently large number of compounds, one can find a molecule for almost any purpose.

We use a large library of peptides (small pieces of protein) as the source of our compounds. During the 1980s, George Smith, now at the University of Missouri, devised a technique for building such a library that employs a phage, a type of virus that infects bacteria (see Figure 2.5). If a short random piece of DNA is inserted into the phage's gene for a surface protein, the phage will thereafter display on its surface a corresponding random peptide. Applying Smith's method, one can create an entire

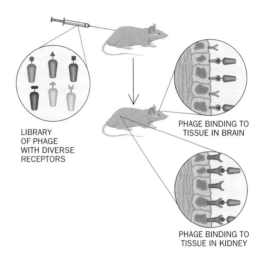

Figure 2.5 PHAGE LIBRARY, consisting of billions of viruses sporting diverse receptor molecules, can help identify the area codes of tissues to which cancer cells home. In one experiment, a phage library was injected into a mouse. Some of the viruses bound uniquely in either the brain or the kidney.

LIBRARY OF PHAGE WITH DIVERSE RECEPTORS

PHAGE BINDING TO TISSUE IN BRAIN

PHAGE BINDING TO TISSUE IN KIDNEY

library of phages carrying a billion different peptides, with each individual phage expressing only one peptide.

Our innovation was to test the affinities of peptides in this library by injecting the diverse viruses into a living animal. Any phage that carried a peptide with an affinity for molecules on a particular tissue would stick there. We looked for and found phages that bound preferentially to blood vessels in a mouse's brain and kidney. That success suggests that specific addresses for other organs could also be discovered and tested for their involvement in tumor cell homing.

Knowledge of the addresses that tumor cells seek may eventually pay off in clinical benefits. Given the vulnerability of tumor cells in transit, anything we can do to make it more difficult for tumor cells to attach to tissues may be beneficial to patients.

Initial work in that direction has started. In 1984 Michael D. Pierschbacher, who was then a postdoctoral associate in my laboratory and is now at Telios Pharmaceuticals, and I showed that all cells attach to fibronectin and several other extracellular matrix proteins at a structure made up of just three amino acids. This result was surprising, given that fibronectin is a long chain of 2,500 amino acids. We went on to show that artificial peptides containing this critical tripeptide (arginine-glycine-aspartic

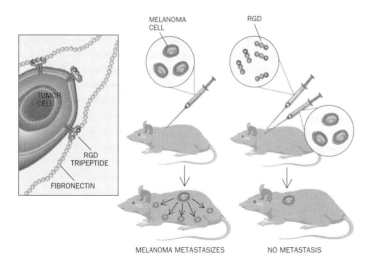

MELANOMA CELL

RGD

TUMOR CELL

RGD TRIPEPTIDE

FIBRONECTIN

MELANOMA METASTASIZES

NO METASTASIS

**Figure 2.6 INHIBITING METASTASIS by interfering with cancer cell adhesion may someday be a therapeutic option. In mouse experiments, injections of RGD, a fragment of the protein fibronectin, discouraged melanoma cells from spreading to the lungs. Presumably, the RGD molecules blocked receptors that wandering cancer cells needed for binding to fibronectin in the extracellular matrix of tissues.**

acid, designated as RGD) can act like a decoy, binding to cells' receptors for fibronectin and blocking their attachment to the matrix.

Martin Humphries and Kenneth M. Yamada, who were then at the National Cancer Institute, and Kenneth Olden, then at Howard University, subsequently showed that if they injected mice with cells from melanomas (lethal skin cancers), RGD peptides could prevent the cells from colonizing the animals' lungs (see Figure 2.6). Such peptides can even prevent metastasis from melanoma tumors grown under the skin of mice—an experimental system that more closely resembles the human disease. David A. Cheresh of the Scripps Research Institute has shown that RGD compounds can also prevent the formation of new blood vessels that nurture tumors. Related compounds therefore may someday augment physicians' anticancer arsenal, but much work will have to be done first so that these peptides can be taken orally and will act longer.

## Understanding Invasion

Disappointingly little is as yet understood in molecular detail about the mechanisms that turn a cancer from a locally growing tumor into a metastatic killer. Some of the same genetic changes that allow cancer cells to escape growth control and avoid apoptosis are clearly important in the early stages of metastatic spread, because they enable cells to survive without anchorage. What then turns on the programs that make the cancer invasive and metastatic, however, is not really known.

Genetic approaches similar to those used in the discovery of oncogenes and tumor suppressor genes have produced some candidates for genes with a specific role in metastasis. Further genetic comparisons of local and metastatic tumors may well explain their differences, but it is also possible that entirely new thinking is needed.

My own bias is that studying resistance to cancer invasion at both the tissue and genetic levels may provide important answers. For example, some tissues are not invaded by cancer: cartilage and, to an extent, the brain. Cancers originating elsewhere in the body can metastasize to the brain, but they do not truly invade the brain tissue—they just grow bigger within and near the blood vessels. Something about brain tissue seems to repel otherwise invasive tumor cells. Some species of animals also appear to be unusually resistant to developing cancers. I suspect that much could be learned if the molecular bases for these and other phenomena were understood. The fact that metastasis is the deadliest aspect of cancer adds the utmost urgency to our quest for this knowledge.

# CAUSES AND PREVENTION

**M**any of the culprits most publicized as causes of cancer actually account for a relatively small fraction of deaths. The good news: we can do more to protect ourselves. And a growing area of study—chemoprevention—is attempting to make the task easier.

# What Causes Cancer?

*The top two causes—tobacco and diet—account for almost two thirds of all cancer deaths and are among the most correctable.*

• • •

Dimitrios Trichopoulos, Frederick P. Li and David J. Hunter

C ancer, a major killer throughout human history, changed its grasp as humankind advanced industrially and technologically. Although the risk of a few types of cancer has declined dramatically in developed countries in this century, the incidence of the most significant forms of the disease has increased. Cancers of the lung, breast, prostate and colon and rectum have all become more frequent in countries where risk factors such as cigarette smoking, unhealthful dietary habits and exposure to dangerous chemicals at work or in the environment are now more common.

As industrialization has proliferated, so, too, have the suspected causes of cancer. In recent years, news accounts have been full of warnings about all manner of modern conveniences, from pharmaceuticals to cellular telephones. Meanwhile the pace of technological advance makes it more vital than ever to single out definitive causes of cancer from an ever expanding array of possibilities.

For this daunting task, researchers rely heavily on epidemiology. Epidemiologists identify factors that are common to cancer victims' history and way of life and evaluate them in the context of current biological understanding. Ultimately, the evidence may persuade researchers that one or more of these factors or characteristics "cause" the disease—that is to say, exposure to them significantly increases the odds of the illness developing.

Over the past half century, epidemiology has enabled researchers not only to ferret out many of the environmental (that is, noninherited) causes of cancer but also to estimate how many annual cancer deaths can be attributed to each one. Although the work cannot be used to predict what will happen to any one individual, it nonetheless provides broadly useful information for people seeking to minimize their exposure to known cancer-causing agents, or carcinogens.

Cancer seems to arise from the effects of two different kinds of carcinogens. One of these categories comprises agents that damage genes involved in controlling cell proliferation and migration. Cancer arises when a single cell accumulates a number of these mutations, usually over many years, and finally escapes from most restraints on proliferation. The mutations allow the cell and its descendants to develop additional alterations and to accumulate in increasingly large numbers, forming a tumor that consists mostly of these abnormal cells. Another category includes agents that do not damage genes but instead selectively enhance the growth of tumor cells or their precursors. The primary danger of malignancies is that they can metastasize, allowing some of their cells to migrate and thus carry the disease to other parts of the body. Finally, the illness can reach and disrupt one of the body's vital organs (see Chapter 1, "How Cancer Arises").

Hardly any researchers doubt that repeatedly exposing parts of the body to, for example, chemicals in tobacco smoke, may eventually bring about the cellular damage that can lead to cancer. But the details of how most exposures give rise to such damage remain elusive. One long-standing theory holds that many environmental stressors, as well as aging and other life processes, play a role by increasing the generation in the body of so-called free radicals—chemically reactive fragments of molecules. By reacting with a gene's DNA, these fragments can damage and permanently mutate the gene. Other cancer-causing agents, such as some viruses, seem to act differently, by accelerating the rate of cell division.

Of course, the genes people inherit from their parents also influence cancer development. Some are born with mutations that directly promote excessive growth of certain cells or the formation of more mutations. Evolutionary pressure, however, assures that such mutations are rare; they are responsible for the development of fewer than 5 percent of fatal cancer cases. (Known genes linked to inherited human cancers are listed in the box "Genes and Cancer Risk.")

On the other hand, more general inherited physiological traits, in contrast to mutations in genes that regulate cell growth, contribute in some way to the vast majority of cancers. For example, inheriting fair skin makes a person more prone to skin cancer. But although fair-skinned people are more susceptible, they develop the disease only after extensive exposure to sunlight, an environmental carcinogen. Further, if someone inherits a normal genetic variant that causes the body to eliminate certain carcinogens relatively inefficiently, that person, after repeated exposure to the carcinogen, will be more likely to acquire the cancer than will a person who has a more efficient form of this gene.

One common question about cancer concerns the number of cases that would be expected to arise naturally in otherwise healthy, genetically normal individuals who somehow had managed to avoid all environmental carcinogens. Only a rough estimate is available, arrived at by comparing populations with very different cancer patterns. Perhaps a quarter of all cancers are "hard core"—in other words, they would develop even in a world free of external influences, simply because of the production of carcinogens within the body and the occurrence of unrepaired genetic mistakes.

Epidemiologists have shown, however, that in most cases, the environment (including lifestyle factors) plays a profound role. How strong are these data? The weak link in cancer epidemiology is the inability to conduct trials in which groups of people, selected at random, are exposed to potential carcinogens or even to potential cancer-preventing compounds. Randomized studies of carcinogens are obviously unacceptable for ethical reasons; unfortunately, lack of such studies can seriously complicate the interpretation of the evidence.

Consequently, we can consider epidemiologic studies to have identified a cause of the disease only when people who have a given type of cancer are consistently found to have a history of unusually high exposure to a particular agent. Alternatively, a link can be declared when a weak relation between an agent and a form of cancer is consistently reported in a variety of circumstances and backed by persuasive biological plausibility.

Accordingly, we have based our assessment of the evidence for what causes cancer either on overwhelming epidemiologic data for which the precise biological mechanisms remain speculative or on weak but consistent epidemiologic findings that are also biologically credible. The role of vegetables and fruits in cancer prevention, for example, tends to be in the former category, whereas the carcinogenic potential of secondhand smoke fits into the latter: relatively few people are afflicted with lung cancer after exposure to secondhand smoke alone, but the connection has been documented consistently and credibly explained.

We have culled the data presented here from hundreds of studies, and the views we offer are shared by many, if not most, researchers and health professionals. In keeping with the standard practice in cancer epidemiology, our focus is on fatal rather than all cancer cases, to avoid distortions introduced by common cancers that only rarely

## Genes and Cancer Risk

Inherited mutations in these genes confer a very high cancer risk. *Red type* indicates cancer most often associated with mutation in the listed gene.

| GENE | TUMORTYPE | GENE CLASS |
|---|---|---|
| *Breast cancer* | | |
| BRCA1 | Breast, ovary | Tumor suppressor |
| BRCA2 | Breast (both sexes) | Tumor supressor |
| p53 | Breast, sarcoma | Tumor suppressor |
| *Colon cancers* | | |
| MSH2 | Colon, endometrium, other | Mismatch repair |
| MLH1 | Colon, endometrium, other | Mismatch repair |
| PMS1,2 | Colon, other | Mismatch repair |
| APC | Colon | Tumor suppressor |
| *Melanoma* | | |
| MTS1 (CDKN2) | Skin, pancreas | Tumor suppressor |
| CDK4 | Skin | Tumor suppressor |
| *Neuroendocrine cancer* | | |
| NF-1 | Brain, other | Tumor suppressor |
| NF-2 | Brain, other | Tumor suppressor |
| RET | Thyroid, other | Oncogene |
| *Kidney cancer* | | |
| WT1 | Wilms' tumor | Tumor suppressor |
| VHL | Kidney, other | Tumor suppressor |
| *Retinoblastoma* | | |
| RB | Retinoblastoma, sarcoma, other | Tumor suppressor |

become lethal. All the results we discuss apply to the United States and to other industrial nations unless we indicate otherwise. The data for developed countries do not necessarily apply to developing countries, in which cancer-causing infections and, increasingly, some occupational carcinogens tend to be more prevalent.

### Tobacco Smoke Is Top Carcinogen

More than half the cancer deaths in the United States—perhaps even 60 percent—can be attributed to tobacco smoke and diet. Smoking causes 30 percent of cancer deaths, making tobacco smoke the single most lethal carcinogen in the United States. Apart from smoking and diet, other environmental factors each contribute to only a few percent of total deaths.

Smoking, mainly of cigarettes, causes cancer of the lung, upper respiratory tract, esophagus, bladder and pancreas and probably of the stomach, liver and kidney. Smoking is implicated in chronic myelocytic leukemia and may also cause cancer of the colon and rectum and other organs. Whether smoking will result in malignancy depends on several factors, including the frequency of smoking, the cigarettes' tar content and—most important— the duration of the habit. Taking up the habit while very young substantially amplifies the risk. The risks vary from one type of cancer to another; thus, on average, smokers are twice as likely to be afflicted with cancer of the bladder but eight times more likely to contract cancer of the lung.

Passive smoking, or inhalation of tobacco smoke in the environment, causes much less lung cancer than active smoking does. Nevertheless, a few thousand people die every year in the United States from cancers attributable mainly to secondhand smoke. Thus, passive smoking is as much a killer as general outdoor air pollution or household exposure to the radioactive gas radon (which is emitted naturally from the earth in some areas).

## Eat Right, Live Longer

Only diet rivals tobacco smoke as a cause of cancer in the United States, accounting for a comparable number of fatalities each year. Animal (saturated) fat in general and red meat in particular are associated with several cancers; both are strongly linked to malignancies of the colon and rectum; saturated fats have been implicated in prostate cancer as well (see Figure 3.1).

A few issues concerning dietary fat still puzzle researchers. Investigations with animals have indicated that under specific conditions certain types of polyunsaturated fat increase the risk for cancer at some bodily sites, but we have little supportive human evidence. Also, rigorous epidemiologic studies have not supported some of the early and still popular hypotheses concerning dietary fat and cancer. For example, high intake of fats (typically, animal fat) in adults has not been shown to increase risk for breast cancer in most investigations that have followed large groups of women for up to a dozen years.

Among nonnutrient food additives, only salt appears to be a significant contributor to cancer. Studies of populations outside the United States suggest that high intake can lead to stomach cancer. Also, in Southeast Asia, very young children who eat a great deal of salty fish tend to have excessive rates of cancer of the nasopharynx (the upper part of the pharynx, which reaches the nasal passages). Similarly, drinking beverages while they are very hot, including maté, a South American tea-like drink, has been shown to increase the risk of esophageal cancer.

In contrast, most investigations of coffee (with or without caffeine) have not linked it to human cancer. Moreover, it does not seem to matter how the beverage is sweetened: there is ample evidence that artificial sweeteners, in reasonable quantities, do not cause cancer.

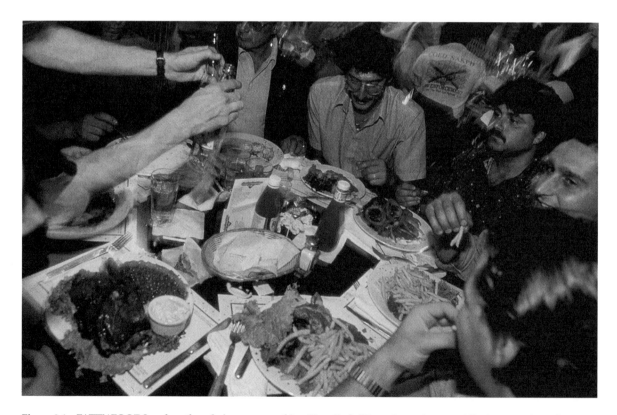

Figure 3.1    FATTY FOODS such as these being consumed in a New York City restaurant can contribute to a variety of cancers.

The links between diet and cancer, however, may have as much to do with what is not in a diet as with what is. Skimping on vegetables and fruits can be a significant contributor to many different kinds of cancer, for reasons that are not fully known. The protective effects of these foods may derive from specific constituents that block the carcinogenic activities of substances made in our own bodies. For instance, antioxidants in foods are believed to neutralize free radicals. Other chemicals in healthful foods, it has been suggested, block the signals that such steroids as estrogen send—signals that cause cells in the breast and elsewhere to proliferate. Yet foods contain thousands of chemicals, and investigators remain unsure of which ones, and which combinations, are most potent as cancer blockers.

Diet can exert its effects not only through the type of calories consumed but also through their quantity. Researchers believe that taking in more energy than is expended can be harmful throughout life, probably through different mechanisms at different ages. Children who overeat and exercise too little often grow more and seem to be at a higher risk of acquiring certain cancers.

These findings have been most striking for breast cancer. Excessive childhood growth, as reflected in attained height and weight, seems to push girls into menstruating when they are relatively young, and early menstruation is a major risk factor for breast cancer (it may contribute to other cancers as well). Such early-life factors as excessive growth caused by overeating and insufficient exercise could be a component cause in perhaps 5 percent of cancers of the breast and prostate, which become fatal relatively frequently.

Obesity in adult life is an important cause of cancer of the endometrium (the lining of the uterus) and an established but relatively weak cause of postmenopausal breast cancer. For unknown reasons, obesity also appears to increase the risk for cancers of the colon, kidney and gallbladder.

Consumption of large quantities of alcoholic beverages, particularly by smokers, increases the risk of cancer of the upper respiratory and digestive tracts, and alcoholic cirrhosis frequently leads to liver cancer. Although modest drinking does seem to reduce the risk of heart disease, converging data suggest that intake of as few as one or two drinks a day may contribute to breast and perhaps colon and rectal cancer.

Alcoholic beverages have been estimated to contribute to about 3 percent (beyond the 30 percent attributed to diet) of total cancer mortality in the developed world. A sedentary way of life contributes to an additional 3 percent. And food additives, mainly salt, may contribute to another 1 percent.

## Radiation and You

Unlike smoking and the dietary practices we have discussed, many other threats, albeit less consequential ones, are rather difficult to avoid. Various forms of radiation—from the sun, electric power lines, household appliances, cellular telephones and naturally occurring, radioactive radon gas—are the most highly publicized of the threats that have been proposed. Radiation causes perhaps 2 percent of all cancer deaths. Most of these fatalities result from natural sources of radiation—the majority can be attributed to melanoma skin cancer triggered by the sun's ultraviolet rays.

Within the ultraviolet spectrum that reaches the earth's surface, the most troubling component consists of the higher-frequency ultraviolet B rays, which can damage DNA. Ultraviolet B rays alone cause more than 90 percent of skin cancers, including melanomas, which are much more frequently fatal than all other forms of skin cancer [see "Sunlight and Skin Cancer," by David J. Leffell and Douglas E. Brash; SCIENTIFIC AMERICAN, July 1996]. Many researchers now believe that the frequency of sunburns during childhood, rather than the cumulative exposure to sunlight, is the key factor in bringing about melanoma. People who tan but do not burn, therefore, are at much less risk.

Another natural source of radiation is radon, a colorless, odorless and radioactive gas that is emitted from the earth in some regions. It can seep into buildings and collect in ground-floor or basement areas. Prolonged breathing of the gas at very high levels, found mostly in underground mines, has been tied to increased incidence of lung cancer. This is not a significant cause of cancer in the general population, however, and radon levels are usually lowered by improving the ventilation of a building or mine.

The electric and magnetic fields generated by power lines and electric household appliances, which oscillate at 60 cycles per second in the United States, are known as extremely low frequency fields. They have been intensively studied for possible cancer-causing effects. So far the collective evidence is confusing, selectively propagated and generally incorrectly perceived. Too often these accounts sow fear by discounting basic science. A cancer-causing genetic mutation cannot be induced by radiation, as far as anyone can discern, unless molecules in the body become charged by gaining or losing one or more electrons—in other words, unless they become ionized. And the photons associated with extremely low frequency fields would have to be a million times more energetic before they could ionize molecules.

Epidemiologic studies have indicated, however, that these fields may somehow increase to a marginal degree the risk of childhood leukemia; the evidence for other cancers is considerably weaker. It is not possible to discount completely the possibility that power lines contribute to some forms of cancer, but the evidence, in our view, is scant. Even for childhood leukemia, the collective evidence is so thin that it can be interpreted either way—as showing a genuine link with the disease or merely as reflecting flaws in the epidemiologic data.

The fear of extremely low frequency fields seems to have several underlying causes. One is the incorrect association made between such fields and other forms of radiation. Another is the wide publicity that has been given to relatively small and preliminary studies.

Radio-frequency electromagnetic radiation, which is emitted by cellular telephones, microwave and other wireless systems and even living creatures, is quite distinct from extremely low frequency fields. Even at the much higher radio frequencies, though, photon energy is still several orders of magnitude below the level required to ionize a molecule. In urban settings, where radio-frequency fields are strongest, ambient energy levels are less than one one-hundredth of those emitted by a human being. Investigators are currently studying the radio emanations associated with cellular telephones for a possible link to brain cancer, but so far no empirical evidence supports such a connection. (The only major study so far did not establish a connection.)

On the other hand, the radiation that comes from nuclear materials and reactions is sufficiently energetic to ionize molecules and is unquestionably carcinogenic. But, again, the general public tends to overestimate the risk posed by low levels of radiation. Among Japanese residents of Hiroshima and Nagasaki who survived longer than approximately one year after the atomic bomb blasts—and who were exposed to radiation levels far higher than most people will ever encounter—only 1 percent have died from cancers known to be related to radiation. Epidemiologic studies have failed to validate claims that the incidence of leukemia is higher among those living near nuclear plants and among children of nuclear reactor workers.

## Of Work, Medications and Microbes

A number of substances now known to be carcinogenic, including asbestos, benzene, formaldehyde, diesel exhaust and radon, were initially revealed to be dangerous in unfortunate "natural experiments" involving exposures to very high concentrations in the workplace (see the box "Carcinogens in the Workplace"). In recent years, however, the control of such occupational carcinogens, at least in the developed world, has brought about a little known success story in public health.

Strict control measures in the workplace over the past 50 years have shrunk the proportion of fatal cancer cases caused by occupational exposures to perhaps less than 5 percent. Before 1950 the proportion may have been twice as great. Unfortunately, though, occupation-associated cancers, which occur mostly in the lung, skin, bladder and the blood-forming (hematopoietic) system, are likely to increase in developing countries as they rapidly industrialize.

Medical treatment, like workplace exposure, has generated unintended insights into cancer causation, as some procedures or medications have turned out to have carcinogenic effects. Ironic as it may seem, medical products and procedures may be responsible for about 1 percent of all cancers. Still, their overall clinical usefulness far outweighs the risks. This is true of many cancer therapies, including radiation and chemotherapy. Some effective drugs or combinations of such drugs used to treat cancers such as Hodgkin's disease can cause acute leukemia in about 5 percent of survivors and, in rare cases, bladder cancer.

Immunosuppressive drugs can also be carcinogenic, causing certain types of lymphomas; supplemental estrogens taken to offset menopausal symptoms have been linked to endometrial and breast cancer. And steroids used for treatment of aplastic anemia have been associated with rare cases of liver cancer.

Early reports indicated that tamoxifen, an experimental breast cancer drug, could occasionally cause endometrial cancer, although recent studies are

# Carcinogens in the Workplace

| CHEMICAL/ PHYSICAL AGENT | CANCER TYPE | EXPOSURE OF GENERAL POPULATION | EXAMPLES OF REQUENTLY EXPOSED OR EXPOSURE SOURCES |
| --- | --- | --- | --- |
| Arsenic | Lung, skin | Rare | Insecticide and herbicide sprayers; tanners; oil refinery workers |
| Asbestos | Mesothelioma, lung | Uncommon | Brake-lining, shipyard, insulation and demolition workers |
| Benzene | Myelogenous leukemia | Common | Painters; distillers and petrochemical workers; dye users; furniture finishers; rubber workers |
| Diesel exhaust | Lung | Common | Railroad and bus-garage workers; truck operators; miners |
| Formaldehyde | Nose, nasopharynx | Rare | Hospital and laboratory workers; manufacture of wood products, paper, textiles, garments and metal products |
| Man-made mineral fibers | Lung | Uncommon | Wall and pipe insulation; duct wrapping |
| Hair dyes | Bladder | Uncommon | Hairdressers and barbers (inadequate evidence for customers) |
| Ionizing radiation | Bone marrow, several others | Common | Nuclear materials; medicinal products and procedures |
| Mineral oils | Skin | Common | Metal machining |
| Nonarsenical pesticides | Lung | Common | Sprayers; agricultural workers |
| Painting materials | Lung | Uncommon | Professional painters |
| Polychlorinated biphenyls | Liver, skin | Uncommon | Heat-transfer and hydraulic fluids and lubricants; inks; adhesives; insecticides |
| Radon (alpha particles) | Lung | Uncommon | Mines; underground structures |
| Soot | Skin | Uncommon | Chimney sweeps and cleaners; bricklayers; insulators; firefighters; heating-unit service workers |

more equivocal. Fertility drugs that mimic the effects of gonadotropins, including Pergonal, are suspected of increasing the risk of ovarian cancer. Growth hormones administered to children might elevate their risk of leukemia. Some diuretics could increase the risk of kidney cancer, and some cholesterol-lowering drugs may heighten the risk of colon and rectal cancer, but for these, too, the evidence is very tenuous.

Oral contraceptives slightly increase the risk of some types of liver tumors and, under certain conditions, of pre-menopausal breast cancer. Yet birth-control pills also reduce the risk of ovarian and endometrial cancer and perhaps that of colon and rectal cancer as well.

Viruses and other infectious agents, overlooked as causes of cancer only 30 years ago, may contribute to about 5 percent of all fatal cases in developed countries (see the box "Microbes That Cause Cancer").

## Pollution's Share

Environmental pollution in the air, water and soil plays an infrequent and difficult-to-document role in human cancer. Harmful effects are hard to verify because they generally result from exposure to several carcinogens at very low levels. Nevertheless, it is reasonable to assume that pollutants could contribute to about 2 percent of fatal cancers, mainly of the lung and bladder.

Ecological studies, which are similar to epidemiologic ones but with less specificity and detail, indicate that lung cancer rates in polluted cities exceed those in rural areas. And, in fact, data do suggest that urban smokers are more likely to develop lung cancer than rural smokers—even after accounting for smoking behavior (how heavily a person smokes, what kind of cigarettes are smoked and so on). Yet urban nonsmokers do not appear to be at increased risk for lung cancer.

Taken together, such studies, emission inventories and chemical analyses of air samples from urban areas suggest that long-term exposure to high levels of air pollution could increase lung cancer risk by about 50 percent, especially among smokers. (Although this figure may seem like a great increase in risk, heavy smoking, by itself, increases risk by about 2,000 percent.) Diesel exhaust, which is probably more carcinogenic than nondiesel exhaust, has been proposed as a likely carcinogenic factor.

Some researchers maintain that organic compounds whose molecules contain chlorine and ring-shaped components increase the risk of breast cancer and, perhaps, other malignancies related to the female hormone estrogen. Among these compounds are ones produced when certain pesticides, such as DDT, have been altered in the body. The underlying hypothesis is that these substances, called xenoestrogens, mimic the body's own (endogenous) estrogens and thus stimulate cell division in the breast and other reproductive organs. The empirical evidence in humans is scant, however, and the estrogenic potency of xenoestrogens is much weaker than that of endogenous estrogens.

Proximity to hazardous-waste sites or contaminated wells may have health effects, but it has not been shown to impart a measurable excess risk for cancer. It is not certain whether the lack of association is genuine or a reflection of the limited capacity of statistical methods to document a very weak correlation.

A few studies have suggested—without convincingly demonstrating—a tenuous positive association between water chlorination and cancer of the bladder. All over the world, but especially in developed countries, chlorination is used to kill germs in drinking water. Even if chlorination did present an extremely small cancer risk—which is by no means certain—the danger would be more than outweighed by chlorine's capacity to prevent the spread of such waterborne diseases as cholera, dysentery and typhoid fever. Investigations of water fluoridation have been reassuring.

## Reproductive and Gynecologic Factors

Among the body's natural processes, those related to reproduction are most closely linked, epidemiologically, to cancer. For women, early age at menarche, late age at first pregnancy and late age at menopause tend to increase the risk for breast cancer; the more offspring a woman has had, the less likely she is to develop cancer of the endometrium, ovary or breast.

Physiological rationales for these observations are elusive, for the most part. No one knows exactly why, for example, early menarche and late menopause are associated with breast cancer. Both may simply extend the period in a woman's life when she is exposed to her own sex hormones, especially estrogen.

# Microbes That Cause Cancer

More than 100 years ago researchers began considering the possibility that cancerous tumors were caused by viruses and other infectious agents. In the decades that followed, though, their attempts to verify this theory failed. Introduction of various infections into animals usually did not yield cancer. Gradually, the theory fell out of favor.

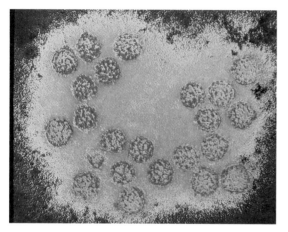

PAPILLOMAVIRUS is a significant cause of cancer.

Over the past 20 years, however, investigators have not only proved that many different types of cancer indeed stem from viruses, bacteria or parasites, they have also learned that perhaps as many as 15 percent of the world's cancer deaths can be traced to them. The vast majority of these cases occur in developing countries, where communicable diseases are much more prevalent. Yet even in such developed countries as the United States, about 5 percent of cancer fatalities result from diseases brought on by infections. Determining exact numbers has been difficult because it often takes several decades for an infection to lead to cancer.

The most common cancer-causing pathogens are the DNA viruses, which propagate by invading the living cells of a host and using the cells' DNA-synthesizing and protein-making machinery to generate copies of themselves. Of these carcinogenic agents, the two most important are the human papillomaviruses types 16 and 18, which are sexually transmitted, and the hepatitis B virus. The papillomaviruses can lead to cancer of the cervix, among other types of cancer, and the hepatitis B virus can cause liver cancer.

Although papillomavirus types 16 and 18 are responsible for 70 to 80 percent of the world's cases of cancer of the genitals and anus, as many as 30 other papillomavirus types may be involved in these cancers, which affect women far more often than men. And in certain places—notably Japan—the hepatitis C virus causes almost as many cases of liver cancer as hepatitis B does. All told, viral infections, mainly hepatitis, cause as many as 80 percent of liver cancer cases around the globe.

Several other viruses have also been found to cause various kinds of cancer, some of which are fairly rare. For instance, Epstein-Barr virus, which is best known for producing mononucleosis, at times becomes carcinogenic as well. It is believed to contribute worldwide to approximately half the cancers of the upper pharynx, as well as to more than 30 percent of all cases of Hodgkin's disease, 10 percent of non-Hodgkin's lymphoma and some gastric cancers. The human immunodeficiency virus (HIV) can cause the soft-tissue cancer known as Kaposi's sarcoma and also lymphoma, a type of cancer characterized by an abnormal proliferation of lymphoid tissue.

*Helicobacter pylori,* the only bacterium linked to cancer, apparently gives rise to the disease in part by causing stomach ulcers [see "The bacteria behind Ulcers," by Martin J. Blaser; SCIENTIFIC AMERICAN, February 1996]. *H. pylori* is strongly associated with the occurrence of stomach cancer, although the proportion of cases attributable to the bacterium remains to be detemined.

Researchers are now trying to understand why these pathogens give rise to cancer in some infected people but not in others. Lately experimental evidence has pointed to secondary occurrences in the body, which can interfere with the host's immune system before an infection becomes cancerous. More knowledge about the details of this chain of events may lead to such new preventive measures as vaccines that block the secondary events, prohibiting a disease from becoming cancerous.

# Why Community Cancer Clusters Are Often Ignored

The 10-foot-long map of Lorraine Pace's Long Island community of West Islip is spread out on her dining-room table. Pace, a 55-year-old breast cancer survivor and the 20th of her neighbors to be diagnosed with the disease, points out patches of yellow-highlighted squares scattered across the map. "These are the breast cancer cases," she explains. Within days of undergoing a lumpectomy in 1992, Pace had galvanized some of the women represented by these squares, and the group—the West Islip Breast Cancer Coalition—spent the next year and a half mapping breast cancer cases in an effort to pinpoint "hot spots" of the disease. They hoped these spots could be correlated with potential environmental threats—and their illness linked to a cause.

At first glance, such community cancer clusters would appear to be the perfect vehicle for identifying cancer-causing agents: by tracing factors to which all the individuals were exposed, investigators should in theory be able to spot a culprit. And the public certainly views clusters that way. State health departments in the United States received about 1,500 requests for cancer cluster investigations in 1989, according to a survey by Daniel Wartenberg of the Robert Wood Johnson Medical School in New Jersey, and that number has continued to increase.

But most cancer clusters appear to happen by chance. It is largely for this reason that health officials these days are usually reluctant to investigate reports of localized excesses in cancer incidence—even the Centers for Disease Control and Prevention gave up routinely investigating cancer clusters in 1990 because they required such intensive resources and yielded so little information in return.

Indeed, although several known carcinogens have been discovered through occupational or medical clusters (for instance, vinyl chloride's link to angiosarcoma in workers who make polyvinyl chloride or the connection of diethylstilbestrol, or DES, to gynecologic cancers in daughters of women who took the drug during pregnancy), only one community cancer cluster has ever been traced to an environmental cause. In that case, researchers linked an epidemic of a rare respiratory cancer called mesothelioma in a Turkish village to an asbestoslike mineral, erionite, that was abundant in the soil.

Among the reasons for which health officials may discount a community's suspicion of common cause is that local groups often lump together different types of cancers (which are unlikely to be triggered by the same carcinogen). These citizens tend to include cases that were diagnosed before the afflicted individuals moved into the neighborhood, or they conduct what the epidemiologist Robert W. Miller of the National Cancer Institute calls epidemiologic gerrymandering: "They find

---

The protective effects of having children early in life, on the other hand, may accrue by causing breast cells to become more differentiated. Differentiation restricts the ability of a cell to grow abnormally, change its type and survive in other types of tissue. A first pregnancy at a young age may differentiate breast cells early in life, after which they would be much less susceptible to carcinogens.

In developed countries, reproductive behavior is determined mainly by social and economic forces. Thus, for educational, career-related and other reasons, millions of women in these countries are putting off childbearing and are also having fewer children, in general, than their mothers and grandmothers did. Unfortunately, such life decisions will lead to higher rates of breast and ovarian cancer. The postponing of first pregnancies by younger women in the United States that has already occurred will increase their breast cancer rates by about 5 to 10 percent within the next 25 years.

Induced abortions have been associated in some studies with a slight increase in breast cancer risk, but the data are not conclusive. Several other associa-

the cases, draw boundaries around the cases, and say, 'Aha, we've found a cluster.'"

Even when such assemblages are ruled out, most clustered cases that initially appear to be statistically significant turn out to be simply naturally occurring spikes in cancer incidence. According to Raymond R. Neutra of the California Department of Health Services, probability theory suggests that 17 percent of the 29,000 towns or census tracts in the U.S. will have at least one of the 80 recognized types of cancer elevated in any given decade, producing 4,930 chance clusters. This high false positive rate is further compounded by the problem of statistical legitimacy—most reported cancer clusters are too small (often fewer than 10 cases) to be judged conclusively.

Even when there is a potential cause in the environment—and a biologically plausible hypothesis of how it might contribute to cancer—trying to trace cancer cases to a specific cause still poses unique challenges. "Cancer cases are clinically nonspecific—you can't look at a leukemia case clinically and say, 'Ah, this is radiation-caused leukemia,'" explains Clark W. Heath of the American Cancer Society. This problem is exacerbated by cancer's latency. Unlike outbreaks of infectious diseases, which can be linked to some recent exposure, a cluster of cancer cases might have its roots in an exposure that occurred 10 to 20 years earlier.

"Reconstructing a person's exposure history is a tremendous scientific challenge," says G. Iris Obrams of the NCI. "For one thing, none of us can reliably recall all the things we've been exposed to. And the further back we go, the more uncertain we are about the accuracy of exposure information and the more likely it is that measurement techniques have changed as well." Obrams also notes that one has to take into account many known cancer risk factors when trying to assess the impact of environmental agents, in part because the disease may be triggered by a combination of environmental, genetic and other factors.

In conducting its own crude version of a cancer cluster investigation, the West Islip Breast Cancer Coalition could never have overcome all these obstacles. But together with many other reports of breast cancer clusters on Long Island, the West Islip situation managed to point epidemiologists in the right direction. Subsequent studies revealed that Long Island did indeed have higher than expected rates of breast cancer incidence and mortality and was, in fact, part of a broad breast cancer cluster extending all the way to Philadelphia. They also helped to establish Long Island as the setting for the largest epidemiologic study ever to be conducted on the link between environmental contaminants and breast cancer.

"We tend to move beyond cluster analysis as quickly as we can," says Obrams, explaining public health officials' decision not to follow up on every reported cluster in Long Island. "We get whatever information we can about clusters to see if there is any lead that we can develop for scientific study, but we know we can get more conclusive data from a larger, well-designed scientific project."

—Lori Miller Kase

tions between cancers of the reproductive tract and certain conditions or behaviors have been noted, but they, too, are not conclusive, are of marginal importance or are thought to be surrogates for actual causes. For example, having multiple sexual partners was once believed to increase a woman's risk of acquiring cancer of the cervix. Instead the increased risk probably reflects greater exposure to sexually transmitted, and potentially carcinogenic, human viruses.

Taking all these considerations into account, we might attribute around 4 percent of cancer deaths to reproduction-related factors.

## Socioeconomic Differences

Differences in cancer rates among socioeconomic groups can usually be attributed to differences in lifestyle. Underprivileged people have higher rates of cancers of the mouth, stomach, lung, cervix and liver and of a type of esophageal cancer (squamous cell cancer). Poverty may be thought of as the underlying cause, because it is almost universally associated with higher rates of tobacco smoking, alcohol consumption, poor nutrition and exposure to certain infectious agents—which, together, can explain most of the cancer-risk propensities listed above.

In contrast, for reasons that remain largely unknown, cancers of the breast, prostate and some other sites are more common among higher socioeconomic groups. Some scientists have speculated that excessive growth in early life, presumably because of reduced physical activity and abundant nourishment, may in some way increase the risk of these cancers. But this hypothesis has not been evaluated rigorously.

Most of the differences in cancer incidence between races, too, can be attributed to socioeconomic factors. Some of the differences between races might have a genetic basis, but genetic variability is higher within than between races. In general, most differences among blacks, whites and Asians can be traced to diet, way of life and environmental exposure. For example, Japanese women in Japan have 25 percent of the risk for breast cancer that white women in the United States have. Yet third-generation Japanese-American women contract breast cancer almost as frequently as other American women do.

## Elusive Mechanisms

Although many of the specific physiological and genetic mechanisms by which environmental carcinogens cause cancer remain elusive, scientists now have a good sense of the extent to which various categories of agents contribute to lethal cancers. By and large, in industrial nations tobacco consumption and dietary habits are the dominant cancer-causing behaviors. In developing nations, cancer cases stemming from infectious agents are more common. But the rapid worldwide spread of the tobacco habit promises to push smoking to the forefront of causes of cancer deaths in these regions, too.

Useful though they are for establishing preventive guidelines and setting health policy objectives, epidemiologic data on the relative significance of environmental carcinogens cannot predict the fate of any given individual. A heavy smoker might avoid lung cancer, a long-term carrier of hepatitis B virus may remain free from liver cancer, and many healthy elderly people have lived long lives on terrible diets. For many of the other factors considered in this chapter, such as ionizing radiation or some occupational factors, only extreme exposures (or carrying mutant genes) put an individual at substantial risk. This is because multiple, interacting factors are almost always necessary for cancer to develop.

At present, we have a very limited understanding of how these interactions allow potential carcinogens to cause cancer. But in time, research may reveal this crucial link, giving us a more complete picture of what cancer is—and how it can be stopped.

# Strategies for Minimizing Cancer Risk

*Simple, realistic preventive measures could save hundreds*
*of thousands of lives every year in developed countries alone.*

• • •

Walter C. Willett, Graham A. Colditz and Nancy E. Mueller

During 1996, more than 550,000 people died of cancer in the United States. In Europe, there were at least 840,000 cancer fatalities. Yet accumulating evidence indicates that in these two parts of the world, which have relatively high and closely tracked cancer mortality rates, more than half these deaths could theoretically have been prevented.

The notion that we can modify cancer risk emerges from decades of investigation. One laboratory experiment after another has demonstrated that a variety of chemicals and other environmental agents can cause cancer in animals, and studies of people have linked heavy exposure to certain substances in the workplace with high risks of specific types of cancer. Also, international studies of migrants repeatedly confirm that they tend to adopt the cancer pattern of their new country within a period that varies from about a decade (for cancer of the colon and rectum) to a few generations (for breast cancer)—a sign that something in the environment, such as changes in diet or exercise patterns, is implicated. If outside factors can increase cancer risk, avoiding those factors should decrease it.

How did we determine the extent to which mortality can be reduced? We began by identifying the lowest rates for various types of cancer among large international populations that keep reliable figures on death from cancer. The incidence of many of the most common cancers in the United States and Europe is much lower in Japan and China. To compile a list of estimated "baseline" cancer incidences, then, we chose the lowest rate for each type of cancer from among the data for the United States, Japan and China. Then we calculated the difference between the highest rate and the baseline. From these comparisons, we conclude that it should be possible to reduce cancer mortality by approximately 60 percent in the United States—perhaps slightly less for black American women, because their incidence rate is already a bit lower. The figures for most Europeans would be similar.

Although we are confident that the death rates of most types of cancer could be substantially cut, there are two notable exceptions. For breast cancer in women and prostate cancer in men, there are no established preventive measures that are likely to have a major impact.

These figures are of interest to more than policy experts and actuaries. For millions of individuals, the results mean that changes in lifestyle can lengthen life—for several years, on average, but several decades for those who would have been stricken in midlife. For most of these people, minimizing the risk of cancer would require a good many changes to address a broad spectrum of causes. For the few people who have inherited mutant genes that dramatically increase the risk of particular types of cancer or for those who have been exposed to unusual occupational hazards, the strategies would be focused mainly on avoiding that specific cancer.

## An Ounce of Prevention

A cancer death can be avoided through prevention of cancer, through detection of the disease early enough to treat it successfully, or through a combination of the two (trying to prevent the disease but being vigilant enough to catch it and treat it early if it develops). Examples of prevention strategies include never smoking and, if it is too late for that, giving up the practice. Kicking the habit enables a former smoker to enjoy a nonsmoker's lower risk for lung cancer after about a decade. Another prevention tactic is eating certain vegetables and other foods that counteract the activity of cancer-causing agents (carcinogens) in the body. In theory, vaccination against the various infectious agents that are known to cause cancer could help as well, although at the moment the only vaccine that can serve this purpose prevents hepatitis B infections.

Early detection relies on the diagnosis of disease at a more treatable stage, before the onset of symptoms that would bring the patient to medical attention (see Chapter 6, "Advances in Cancer Detection"). This approach has been applied to some cancers, such as cervical and colorectal cancer. Epidemiologic studies indicate that death rates from these two diseases could be reduced by at least 50 percent if screening were widely applied, making it possible to remove precancerous growths and to detect malignancies earlier. The test for cervical cancer is the well-known Pap smear; the most effective procedures for detecting cancer of the colon and rectum are sigmoidoscopy and colonoscopy.

No matter how effective they may be, early detection and treatment are less desirable than primary prevention, for many reasons. Most obviously, prevention avoids the shock and pain of being diagnosed and treated for cancer. In addition, many methods for cancer prevention, such as regular exercise and a sensible diet, have side benefits, such as reducing the risk of cardiovascular and other diseases—which makes them even more cost-effective in comparison with treatment. Moreover, the ability of medical science to treat many forms of cancer is limited by the disease's tendency to spread to other parts of the body, the phenomenon of metastasis. And of course, the failure of prevention still leaves treatment as a last resort.

These advantages notwithstanding, the power of prevention as a defense against cancer has never been fully appreciated by the public at large, if the widespread persistence of unhealthy habits is any indication. This disappointing observation is perhaps understandable. It is, after all, impossible to tell whether a healthy lifestyle warded off cancer in an individual. Conversely, successful treatment invariably becomes a landmark event. Moreover, the results of effective treatment become apparent quickly, whereas the impact of a prevention regime—quitting smoking, say—may take years to emerge.

As in Chapter 3, "What Causes Cancer," we focus here on fatal kinds of cancer rather than all cases to avoid distortions introduced by the large number of highly localized cancers and those forms of skin cancer that are seldom fatal. For each major cause, we estimate how much mortality could be reduced for people living in the U.S. or a similar developed country.

## Potent Mix: Tobacco and Alcohol

Most cancer prevention campaigns rightly focus on controlling the tobacco smoking epidemic. But the goal has proved to be an elusive one. The decline of smoking in most developed countries has been more than offset in recent years by a rapid increase elsewhere in the world. Small-scale programs and traditional health education efforts are no match for the addictive power of nicotine and the marketing clout of the tobacco industry.

In democratic societies, three complementary approaches appear most promising: improved general education, taxation, and cultivation of an anti-smoking social ethos. The strong inverse association between educational achievement and smoking reinforces the importance of health education for all segments of society. High taxes on tobacco products, as well as social disapproval or regulation of smoking in office buildings, airplanes and public places, have been shown to reduce smoking rates.

Perhaps, too, we could do more to bring people's perceptions of risk in line with reality. It is not uncommon to meet heavy smokers who are genuinely concerned about the health effects of unproved or possibly trivial environmental agents, such as magnetic fields or chlorinated water.

Tobacco smoking cannot be completely eradicated; hardly any vices ever have been. But on the basis of the dramatic decline in smoking among the more educated adults in the United States over the past few decades and the increasingly pervasive sentiments against smoking, it would not be unrealistic to hope that tobacco smoking—and, eventually, deaths related to tobacco—can be reduced by about two thirds within a few decades. Such a reduction would of course require that the trend not only continue but also spread to less educated groups.

The moderate intake of alcoholic beverages, at about one or two a day, reduces mortality from cardiovascular causes. At the same time, alcohol has been linked with several forms of cancer. Effects of alcohol consumption and tobacco smoking are also believed to interact to cause cancer in the upper respiratory and gastrointestinal tracts.

Clearly, on many grounds, heavy alcohol consumption should be avoided. Anyone considering drinking moderately for the good of the heart should consult a physician and take into account any family history of alcoholism while weighing the risk of cancer against that of cardiovascular disease. Also, for women younger than 50 years, who are at relatively low risk of cardiovascular disease, there does not appear to be any reduction in mortality from moderate alcohol use.

Overall, alcohol-related cancer mortality could probably be decreased by about one third if a realistically smaller number of people had more than two drinks a day.

## Preventing Diet-Related Cancer

Although we know little about the specific beneficial or harmful constituents of food, we have a good idea of what people should eat if they want to improve their odds of avoiding cancer. Their diet should be high in vegetables, fruits and legumes (such as peas and beans) and low in red meat, saturated fat, salt and sugar. Carbohydrates should be consumed as whole grains—whole-wheat bread and brown rice as opposed to white bread and rice,

for example. Added fats should come mainly from plants and should be unhydrogenated; olive oil, especially, appears potentially beneficial.

Everyone should work assiduously to avoid being overweight, ideally in part through physical activity (see Figure 4.1). In addition to helping to control weight, exercise reduces the incidence of colon cancer and, perhaps, of other types as well. Regular physical activity during childhood and adolescence may also slow down excessive growth and avoid an early onset of menstrual cycles, both of which have been implicated in malignancy.

Some evidence links increased risk of breast and prostate cancer with high birth weight and other factors dating to around the time of birth. Although this information is of interest to scientists, it does not readily translate into practical means of prevention. This situation contrasts with that in most other forms of cancer, for which prevention strategies became apparent when causes were established. The implication is that in the near future, in developed countries, the incidence of cancers of the breast and prostate will prove more difficult to reduce—and that, therefore, these cancers could be responsible for an increasing percentage of all cancer mortality as deaths from many other kinds of cancer decline (see Figures 4.2 and 4.3).

Although the benefits of exercise and dietary moderation have been known for decades, the proportion of overweight Americans has been increasing. Between 1980 and 1991 the prevalence of obesity rose by 33 percent in the United States. Nevertheless, many people, particularly those with higher education and income, have learned how to avoid age-related weight gain, so it is not unrealistic to hope for some improvement among other groups in the foreseeable future.

Similarly, modest shifts toward more healthy habits by the population as a whole should be possible. If a majority of people were to make two or more wise changes—exercising vigorously for 20 minutes a day, eating one more serving of leafy vegetables each day or consuming no more than one serving of red meat a week, for example—both diet-related and sedentary-life-related cancer mortality might be reduced by about one quarter. Taken together, such changes could prevent an estimated 40,000 premature cancer deaths annually in the United States. The same measures would also lessen the incidence of cardiovascular disease, saving additional lives. Further knowledge of the specific cancer-fighting components of vegetables and fruits, which

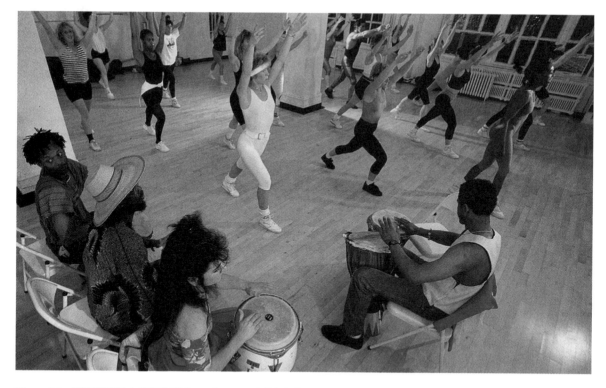

Figure 4.1  **PHYSICAL ACTIVITY throughout one's life helps to ward off several types of cancer.**

scientists are now striving to uncover, could allow more focused and effective dietary strategies (see Chapter 5, "Chemoprevention of Cancer").

A great deal of evidence already suggests that most Americans do not get enough folic acid in their diets. Lack of this nutrient may contribute to colon cancer and heart disease, so multivitamins that include folic acid, also called folate, might prove beneficial. Regarding so-called megavitamins, little reliable research indicates that these highly concentrated supplements are any more protective against cancer than plain old multivitamins (and even for these, a benefit has not been established).

## Avoiding Viruses

The human papillomavirus is the most common cancer-causing infection in the United States. The sexually transmitted strains, which can lead to cervical cancer, are the most lethal. They can be combated, however, by the same measures directed against transmission of the AIDS-causing human immunodeficiency virus (HIV)—such as delaying initial sexual activity, reducing casual sexual con-

tact and using latex condoms. More widespread application of these precautions could lead to a further modest decline in deaths from cervical cancer and from other genital tumors traceable to papillomavirus. Pap screening, which enables doctors to detect incipient tumors early enough to cure them, has contributed over the past few decades to the dramatic decline in deaths from cervical cancer. Greater use of this technique could enhance this decrease.

In the United States, the hepatitis B and C viruses cause a minority of the cases of hepatocellular carcinoma, a form of liver cancer. The recently introduced vaccines against the hepatitis B virus, improved screening of blood and blood products and more pervasive use of disposable syringes and needles by intravenous drug abusers are all expected to help reduce the spread of the viruses. Although common, the Epstein-Barr virus causes relatively few American cancer deaths. No immunization for this large, complex virus is available yet.

Mortality from stomach cancer in the United States has been declining for the past half century.

## Women's Probability of Acquiring Cancer by Age 75

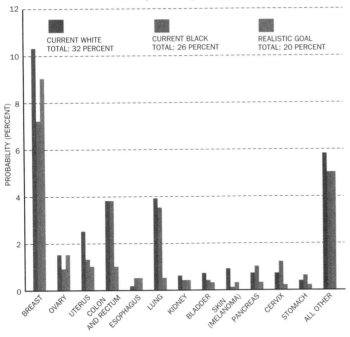

Figure 4.2 REALISTIC GOAL for reducing the chances of being stricken with any kind of cancer during a normal life span is, for white women, about one third. The corresponding goal for black women is less because their rates are already lower than those of white women.

## Men's Probability of Acquiring Cancer by Age 75

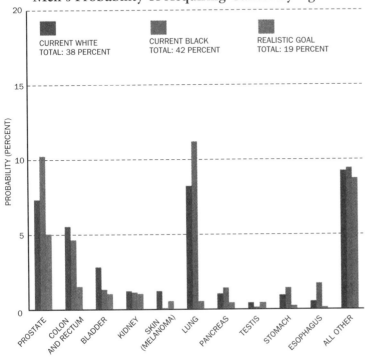

Figure 4.3 MEN SHOULD BE able to cut their risk of acquiring cancer at least in half. Almost anyone can achieve such a reduction in cancer risk by adopting prudent habits, such as not smoking, exercising regularly, eating plenty of fruits, vegetables and whole grains and by avoiding animal fats, red meat, refined starches and alcohol. That such reductions in risk are realistic is supported by the fact that they have already been largely achieved by Seventh-Day Adventists, many of whom follow these practices.

A partial explanation may be that improved sanitation has delayed infection by Helicobacter pylori, a bacterium causing chronic stomach inflammation that can become cancerous. Later infection by this prevalent microbe gives the disease less time to develop. Also, people now tend to consume less salt and more fruits and vegetables that contain vitamin C than was common years ago; these dietary improvements also seem to interfere with the infection's ability to induce cancer. Use of antibiotics to treat the infection may lead to further reductions.

Barring a breakdown of the measures and policies currently in force, mortality from cancers of infectious origin is likely to decline over the next few decades in the United States, and most other advanced countries, probably by about one fifth. In less developed countries, however, infections are likely to continue causing substantial cancer deaths.

## Reproductive Factors

Considerable evidence links certain reproductive behavior with cancer, particularly for cancer of the breast or ovaries in women. Unfortunately, as with many other findings about the causes of breast cancer, the insights have not led to effective prevention strategies. Part of the problem is that reproductive behavior is driven mainly by social and economic forces, so that modifying it to prevent cancer is for the most part unrealistic.

Birth-control pills cause a small increase in breast cancer rates while they are being used, but this excess risk declines rapidly after their use is discontinued. Use before 35 years of age, when the incidence of breast cancer is low, has minimal impact on breast cancer mortality. On the other hand, use of oral contraceptives for five or more years substantially reduces the lifetime risk of ovarian and endometrial cancer. Thus, the overall impact on cancer mortality—if pill use is limited to earlier reproductive life—is beneficial. Some evidence suggests that tubal ligation may also reduce ovarian cancer risk but that vasectomy may increase risk of prostate cancer in men.

Hormonal contraceptives that simulate early pregnancy in women in their teens or early twenties—or an early menopause in women in their thirties or forties—could potentially reduce the risks for breast cancer. A modest amount of research and development is being done on such contraceptives.

Although the first early-menopause preparations may be available within a decade, another 10 years or more may be needed for investigators to assess their effects on breast cancer risk.

## Environment and Pollution

Over the past 20 years, no field of cancer epidemiology has seen as many new hypotheses as that concerned with environmental pollution. The candidate carcinogens are diverse enough to include extremely low frequency magnetic fields from electric power lines, radio-frequency electromagnetic radiation used in cellular telephones, proximity to nuclear plants or chemical-waste dumps, water fluoridation and even unseen, unspecified sources responsible for "clusters" of cancer cases within small geographic regions. Few of these hypotheses have been corroborated. But they all serve an important function: preserving the necessary vigilance in the face of the exploding pace of technological change.

With respect to radiation from nuclear or x-ray sources and workplace carcinogens, all any one citizen can do is demand that the authorities enforce regulations. Technological progress resulting in a shift away from traditional industrial employment, fewer workers in relatively high cancer risk jobs, and the phasing out of asbestos use in buildings justify an expectation that deaths from job-related cancers can be cut by about one half over the next several decades.

In addition, greater awareness of the risks of being in the sun between 11 A.M. and 3 P.M. and more widespread use of sunscreens could reduce deaths from melanoma, the most lethal form of skin cancer, by one half. The reduction will be less, however, if the depletion of the earth's ozone layer continues, allowing more of the sun's ultraviolet rays through. Part of the ultraviolet spectrum is responsible for most skin cancers.

Air pollution has declined over the past 30 years in the United States. Although the measures that brought about the reduction were mostly aimed at short-term goals, such as providing relief for those suffering from asthma, some drop in pollution-related cancer mortality may occur. Yet any such benefit will be as difficult to document as the existence of the original link itself. A decline of one quarter in pollution-related cancer, corresponding to less than 1 percent of all cancer deaths, may be possible.

Mammography, menopausal estrogens and tamoxifen for preventing breast cancer have also come under scrutiny as possible cancer-causing agents. It is now generally recognized that mammography conveys a negligible risk and a substantial benefit. Menopausal estrogens can cause cancer of the endometrium and the breast, although preparations that include progestin are safer in relation to endometrial cancer.

Tamoxifen, a valuable drug for treating breast cancer, is now being evaluated to determine whether it can prevent breast cancer among healthy women who are at high risk for the disease. The catch is that considerable evidence indicates that tamoxifen can cause endometrial cancer. No doubt, medical products and procedures will continue to cause a small proportion of all cancers, but in general, their substantial benefits outweigh their risks.

## What to Do

In sum, anyone can reduce his or her chances of being afflicted with cancer by following some sensible guidelines: eat plenty of vegetables and fruits; exercise regularly and avoid weight gain; and avoid tobacco smoke, animal fats and red meats, excessive alcohol consumption, the midday sun, risky sexual practices and known carcinogens in the environment or workplace. Of course, not everyone will follow this advice, and many others will not heed it consistently. Taking this reality into account, we estimate (see Figure 4.4) that a reasonable medium-term objective of prevention programs in the United States or any other economically advantaged population is a reduction of cancer mortality by about one third, even without new discoveries or technological developments. This reduction is far less than

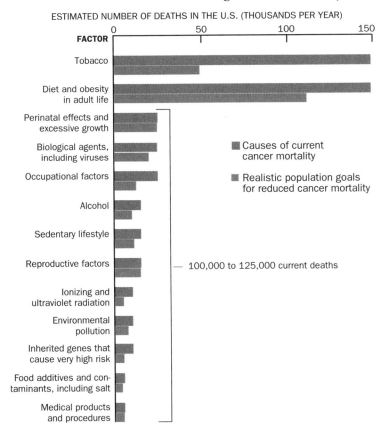

### Realistic Goals for Reducing Cancer Mortality

Figure 4.4  **TOBACCO AND DIET, including the latter's effects on obesity, account for about 300,000 cancer fatalities every year in the U.S.—or about 60 percent of the country's annual cancer mortality. Researchers hope these numbers, particularly those for tobacco-caused cancer deaths, can be significantly reduced. Other factors, however, such as those dating to around the time of birth (perinatal factors) or those related to reproduction, are expected to be much more resistant to improvement.**

the almost two thirds that is theoretically possible, but it is still considerable. With further research and new information about the causes of cancer, more reductions are likely.

For a small group of people, prevention strategies will be much more customized. Individuals born with mutant genes for various cancers, which greatly increase the probability that they will be afflicted, are commonly offered genetic counseling that focuses on preventing the kind of cancer they are facing. Assuming that such mutations are uncommon, that some high-risk births might be avoided and that prophylactic measures are taken in affected persons, it might be possible to reduce mortality from inherited cancer by about one half. Still, this is a very speculative estimate in a field that is rapidly changing and in which any impact would not be measurable for many years.

Because most of the actions to prevent cancer must be taken by individuals, the distribution of accurate information, together with peer support for the elimination of bad habits and for other behavioral changes, is critical. But effective cancer prevention requires activities at other levels, too, including counseling and screening by health care providers. At this level, dissemination of scientifically sound information to the providers themselves is crucial.

Another level involves regulation by government agencies to minimize the public's exposure to harmful agents, promote healthier products and ensure that industry provides safe working environments. In some cases, officials will have to deal with the displacement of workers whose livelihood depends on the production of toxic products. For example, the costs of subsidizing tobacco farmers to grow something other than tobacco may help avoid higher costs in the future if fewer people need to be treated for lung cancer. An additional level involves the implementation of policies to improve public health. Examples include providing community facilities for safe physical activity, such as bikeways for commuting and after-school gymnasium programs for children.

At the international level, the actions of developed countries affect cancer prevention worldwide. Unfortunately, tobacco exports are often promoted, and hazardous manufacturing processes are moved to unregulated Third World countries. Both trends will contribute to rising rates of cancers worldwide.

Most types of cancer are to a large extent preventable, even with today's knowledge and technologies. The "war on cancer," primarily fought by searching for improved cancer treatments, has met with limited success and should be better balanced by more extensive efforts in prevention.

# Chemoprevention of Cancer

*Someday people should be able to avoid cancer or
delay its onset by taking specially formulated pills or foods.*

• • •

Peter Greenwald

For many years now, scientists have understood that the onset of cancer is a gradual, stepwise process that may unfold over the course of decades, rather than a single, fixed event that can be dated in a pathologist's report. Carcinogenesis encompasses a prolonged accumulation of injuries at several different biological levels and includes both genetic and biochemical changes in cells. At each of these levels there is an opportunity for intervention—a chance to prevent, slow or even halt the gradual march of healthy cells toward malignancy.

Chemoprevention is the attempt to use natural and synthetic compounds to intervene in the early precancerous stages of carcinogenesis, before invasive disease begins. The idea behind such intervention is simple. Certain foods, including many vegetables, fruits and grains, offer protection against various cancers. Chemoprevention researchers try to find substances—either components of food or pharmaceuticals—that can prevent or halt carcinogenesis. Their goal is to use these substances in pills or in modified foods, as a prevention strategy for people at high risk for cancer—much as drugs that reduce cholesterol, blood pressure and clotting of the blood benefit people at high risk for heart disease and stroke.

The endeavor began in the mid-1950s, when investigators first directed their knowledge of carcinogenesis toward a search for substances that could inhibit tumor formation. This approach to cancer prevention was named "chemoprevention" in the mid-1970s by Michael B. Sporn, an innovator in cancer prevention research (see the box "A Plea for Prevention"). Since that time, researchers have identified hundreds of potential chemopreventive agents through animal research and cancer epidemiology (the study of specific groups of people, such as ethnic groups and postmenopausal women, to identify factors related to cancer incidence) and sometimes from studies of the medical treatments. More than two dozen of those chemopreventive agents are now being tested on people.

The quest for chemopreventive compounds, however, entails overcoming significant obstacles. For example, those who plan clinical trials of chemopreventive preparations face a constraint that is absent in trials of chemical therapies for disease. The criteria for selecting agents to be used in chemoprevention must be quite different from

# A Plea for Prevention

Michael B. Sporn, professor of pharmacology and medicine at Dartmouth Medical School, has argued repeatedly, in print and at the podium, that an "obsession" with curing advanced disease has blinded cancer researchers to the promise of prevention. Like heart disease, he says, cancer is the culmination of years of subtle pathology. It is never too soon to intervene—but it is often too late.

"The concept that people with cancer were healthy until a doctor told them that they've got an invasive lesion makes no sense at all," Sporn says. "And nobody in the oncology community is doing anything to change that viewpoint—except for a few believers in chemoprevention."

Sporn is among the most prominent of chemopreventionists, who seek to develop substances that can block the onset of cancer. He led the National Cancer Institute's laboratory of chemoprevention from its inception in 1978 until 1995, when he moved to Dartmouth. And he pioneered chemoprevention research in the mid-1970s with laboratory studies of retinoids, vitamin A analogues that can inhibit tumor development. Noting the success of cardiovascular intervention strategies in reducing deaths from heart disease, he has long called for a revision in cancer research priorities that would emphasize the disease's beginnings rather than its terminal stages.

"We haven't wanted to deal with precancerous states, because there's been nothing you could do about them," Sporn states. But he is confident that this predicament will change, if enough resources are brought to bear on it. The ideal result, he speculates, would be one or several nontoxic, low-cost chemopreventive agents that could be supplied universally, like fluoride in drinking water—easy pills to swallow.

—Karen Wright

those used in chemotherapy because chemotherapeutic agents are often chosen for their ability to kill cells; they harm cancer cells more than healthy ones but can still be quite toxic and thus produce troubling side effects. In contrast, chemopreventive agents must be nontoxic and relatively free of side effects, because they are meant to be administered to healthy people for long periods. Thus, agents will be formulated to be taken orally, as pills or as foods or beverages modified to increase their protective constituents.

Furthermore, to be most effective, chemopreventive agents must be used within a broad context of prevention. Like cardioprevention programs, a preventive program for cancer would include sophisticated evaluation of a patient's risk, as well as recommendations for lifestyle changes. Many experts believe such programs could ultimately be among the most effective ways of reducing cancer mortality.

## Vital Vegetables

Food is a source of some of the most promising chemopreventive compounds. Vegetables and fruits are likely to decrease cancer risk, but isolating the effects of individual food constituents has proved difficult. Nevertheless, investigations of so-called phytochemicals ("plant chemicals"), pioneered by Lee W. Wattenberg of the University of Minnesota, have identified many agents that protect against cancer in laboratory studies. They include such vitamins as A (and its analogues), C and E, as well as compounds without nutritional value, such as indoles, isothiocyanates, dithiolthiones and organosulfur compounds.

Dithiolthiones, for example, are potential chemopreventive agents found in cruciferous vegetables such as broccoli, cauliflower and cabbage. A synthetic dithiolthione called Oltipraz has been shown to inhibit the development of tumors of the lung, colon, mammary glands and bladder in laboratory animals (see Figure 5.1). Like a number of other beneficial substances, Oltipraz interferes with carcinogenesis in more than one way. For example, it activates liver enzymes that can detoxify carcinogens in the bloodstream. This effect may be related to the activity of dithiolthiones in cruciferous vegetables, which, along with other dithiolthiones, are thought to activate enzymes that produce natural pesticides that ward off or kill insects.

A host of chemicals derived from plants have demonstrated chemopreventive potential in the

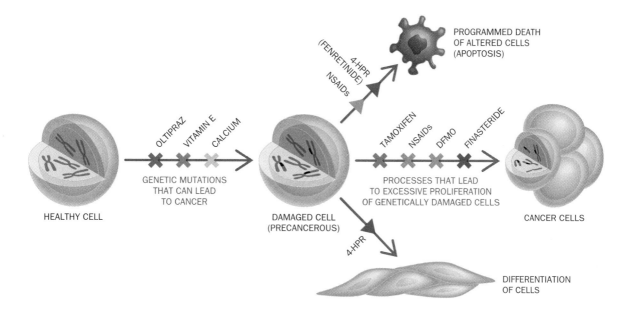

Figure 5.1  **PROGRESSION TO CANCER can be avoided in two basic ways. Some chemopreventive supplements** (*represented by colored Xs*), **are intended to halt the progression, either before or after genetic mutations cause a cell to become precancerous. Another approach** relies on agents (*shown as colored triangles*) that divert the progression to a benign outcome, such as the death or differentiation of precancerous cells (differentiation steers affected cells back toward their normal, noncancerous state).

laboratory. Sulforaphane, an isothiocyanate, is also thought to work by activating detoxifying enzymes in the liver. Isolated from broccoli, sulforaphane is one of the chemicals responsible for the sharp taste of raw cruciferous vegetables. In rats, it blocks the formation of chemically induced mammary tumors. Adding soy to a rodent's diet also decreases the incidence of mammary tumors in rodents. Genistein, a compound in soy, may be one of several specific compounds responsible for that protection. It seems to prevent cancer through multiple mechanisms, among them the inhibition of angiogenesis—the formation of new blood vessels essential for the growth and spread of tumors.

Tea extracts show chemopreventive effects in animals as well. Researchers believe the principal chemopreventive agent in the extracts is epigallocatechin gallate, an antioxidant that accounts for about 50 percent of the solid materials in brewed green tea. Laboratory studies at the American Health Foundation in Valhalla, N.Y., are suggesting similar benefits from black tea.

## Surprising Trials

Cancer researchers have screened hundreds of plant compounds to identify candidates for chemoprevention such as those mentioned; they must systematically and carefully evaluate voluminous evidence from laboratory experiments and epidemiologic studies to determine which of those compounds might be most beneficial for humans. A chosen few have already advanced to the next stage in evaluation: a clinical trial with human subjects. And some of those trials have yielded surprising results.

Beginning in 1985, for example, beta-carotene was included in two large, long-term chemoprevention trials sponsored by the National Cancer Institute: the Alpha-Tocopherol, Beta-Carotene Lung Cancer Prevention Study (ATBC) (see the box "Some Clinical Chemoprevention Trials"), conducted with Finnish subjects and scientists, and the Beta-Carotene and Retinol Efficacy Trial. In these studies, daily doses of beta-carotene and either vitamin E (alpha-tocopherol) or vitamin A (retinol) were

# Some Clinical Chemoprevention Trials

A variety of drug, vitamin and mineral supplements have been tested for their ability to lower the dangers of cancer in populations at risk. Some of these chemoprevention protocols show promise, but others seem to be actively harmful or have not yet shown clear benefit. A few of the past and ongoing trials conducted by the National Cancer Institute are described below.

## ALPHA-TOCOPHEROL, BETA-CAROTENE LUNG CANCER PREVENTION STUDY (ATBC)

*Would daily oral doses of alpha-tocopherol (vitamin E) or beta-carotene, or both, reduce rates of lung and other cancers in male smokers?*

**Tested on:** 29,133 male smokers for five to eight years (beginning in 1985)

**Findings:** ▲ 18 percent increase in lung cancer in beta-carotene group

▼ 34 percent decrease in prostate cancer in vitamin E group

● Small but statistically insignificant decrease in colorectalcancer in vitamin E group

## ISOTRETINOIN EFFICACY TRIAL

*Would daily oral doses of the retinoid isotretinoin reduce rates of secondary tumors in high-risk people who have been initially treated for head and neck cancer?*

**Tested on:** 100 cancer-free, high-risk people for one year (beginning in 1983)

**Findings:** ▼ 83 percent decrease in secondary tumors

## LINXIAN GENERAL POPULATION TRIAL

*Would daily oral doses of four combinations of vitamins and minerals reduce rates of esophageal and stomach cancer in high-risk people in China?*

**Tested on:** 29,584 people for six years (beginning in 1985)

**Findings:** ▼ 21 percent decrease in stomach cancer deaths for people taking beta-carotene, vitamin E and selenium; follow-up studies are ongoing

## BREAST CANCER PREVENTION TRIAL (BCPT)

*Would daily oral doses of the drug tamoxifen reduce rates of breast cancer in women at high risk or older than 35 years?*

**Tested on:** 16,000 women for five years (beginning in 1992)

**Findings:** ● Study is ongoing; no results yet available

---

administered for several years to tens of thousands of people at high risk for lung cancer. Epidemiologic evidence linking dietary levels of beta-carotene to reduced cancer risk had strongly supported the studies' hypothesis, namely, that administering the nutrients would protect against lung cancer.

Instead the rate of lung cancer in cigarette smokers taking beta-carotene increased slightly in both trials. Scientists have no ready explanation for the increase, but it seems likely that substances other than beta-carotene are responsible for the protective effects of vegetables and fruits. A long-term study of 22,000 U.S. physicians showed no evidence of harm or benefit from taking beta-carotene.

Also surprising in the ATBC study was the fact that the men who received doses of vitamin E (alone or with beta-carotene) experienced 34 percent fewer cases of prostate cancer and 16 percent fewer cases of colon and rectal cancer than their peers, whereas their rates of lung cancer were unaffected. This finding has not been confirmed, however, and the ATBC study was not designed to examine these correlations. The apparent decrease in prostate and colon and rectal cancers could either be a benefit of the vitamin E doses or just a chance occurrence. More trials are needed to explore this intriguing connection. Results from the two beta-carotene studies clearly illustrate the importance of human trials both in testing established hypotheses about chemoprevention and in generating new ones.

## Promising Preventive Treatments

Vitamins and food-derived compounds are the focus of a large part of chemopreventive research, but a number of drugs being used for treatment may also be suitable for prevention. One such drug is tamoxifen, the antiestrogen medication that has demonstrated great potency in the treatment of breast cancer. First synthesized in 1966 for birth-control research, tamoxifen is thought to thwart cancer by blocking estrogen receptors that, when occupied, stimulate cell proliferation.

An ongoing, 10-year study by a national collaborative group of U.S. physicians and scientists—headquartered in Pittsburgh—and the National Cancer Institute is testing tamoxifen's ability to prevent breast cancer in thousands of healthy women who are at increased risk for the disease. In earlier studies of breast cancer patients, tamoxifen reduced the incidence of new tumors in the unaffected breast by about 40 percent. Those figures provided the rationale for investigating tamoxifen as a preventive agent. But although it has clearly been a boon to breast cancer patients, tamoxifen has side effects, the most serious of which are increased risks of uterine cancer and blood-clot formation. Because of those risks, some women's health advocates have questioned the use of the compound by healthy women for prevention.

Yet the knowledge gained from a large-scale preventive trial of tamoxifen could help researchers understand how to synthesize a second generation of antiestrogen drugs having greater potency and fewer risks than those associated with tamoxifen itself.

Retinoids, derived from vitamin A, also have been tested in treatment studies and can slow or prevent the development of many epithelial cancers, particularly those of the head and neck.

Retinoids probably work by encouraging cell maturation and specialization, processes that essentially force cells to forsake proliferation. Over the past decade, researchers at the M. D. Anderson Cancer Center in Houston have conducted a careful series of chemoprevention trials using a synthetic retinoid called isotretinoin. In part because of the compound's toxicity, these trials have been confined to high-risk individuals: heavy smokers or drinkers who already have or have had head or neck tumors and who therefore have a good chance of developing more malignancies. For these people, the potential benefits of chemoprevention clearly outweigh the known disadvantages.

## Many Trials Ahead

Over the next decade, numerous trials of potential chemopreventive agents will deepen our understanding of the mechanisms and practical benefits of chemoprevention. A synthetic compound called difluoromethylornithine (DFMO), for example, is being tested in groups of 40 to 120 people for the prevention of many different types of cancer, including breast, cervical, prostate, bladder, colon and skin. DFMO interferes with the activity of an enzyme (ornithine decarboxylase) essential for cell proliferation. Nonsteroidal anti-inflammatory drugs (NSAIDs) such as aspirin and ibuprofen seem to inhibit this same enzyme and are also being studied in small chemoprevention trials for colon cancer. In general, these anti-inflammatories protect the body from disease in a number of ways that go beyond inhibiting cell proliferation. But prolonged use of NSAIDs may cause gastrointestinal side effects, such as bleeding or ulcers.

The "gold standard" of chemoprevention trials is still the large, prospective study, which monitors future development of disease in either high-risk individuals or the general population. In these trials, the experimental agent may need to be administered for many years, after which a number of years are required to assess the effects fully. One such trial now under way is examining the ability of finasteride to prevent prostate cancer. Finasteride, which is already used to treat benign enlargement of the prostate, inhibits the conversion of testosterone in the prostate to a more potent androgen that is thought to promote cancer. In the Prostate Cancer Prevention Trial, finasteride or a placebo is being given daily to 18,000 men for seven years; follow-up could take a decade or more.

To help speed results of prospective chemoprevention trials, researchers are investigating the use of biomarkers as surrogate measures of a compound's success. Biomarkers are physiological manifestations of changes that may occur on the pathway to cancer; if an intervention reduces the incidence of these signs in a population, chances are that the agent will lower the incidence of cancer as well. Ongoing trials of chemopreventive agents for colon cancer, for example, will determine the efficacy of calcium, NSAIDs and other compounds based on the incidence of intestinal polyps, a benign precursor to colon cancer, rather than the incidence of the cancer itself. Other biomarkers under investigation include specific genetic mutations, altered levels or forms of certain proteins in blood serum and urine, and tissue pathologies such as precancerous lesions.

Biomarkers could also aid physicians in evaluating a patient's risk of acquiring cancer, much as blood lipid levels are used in standard medical practice to monitor heart disease risk. Such evaluations will be an integral part of future chemoprevention programs.

Informed by such profiles, physicians could tailor to each patient a chemopreventive strategy that would stall carcinogenesis long before it progressed to invasive disease. The power of this approach is sure to grow as researchers continue to identify promising new chemoprevention agents and clinical trials begin to provide insight into these substances' effects in humans. With the advance of these investigations and our greater understanding of cancer, chemoprevention will undoubtedly play a major role in reducing cancer incidence as well as the number of deaths caused by the disease.

# Current Controversy: Is Hormone Replacement Therapy a Risk?

• • •

Nancy E. Davidson

Thanks to advances in public health and medicine, the average American woman will be postmenopausal for about one third of her life. As a result, she will ultimately need to make a decision about hormone replacement therapy. During the 1960s, doctors began to prescribe a short-term regimen of estrogen to control menopausal symptoms such as hot flashes and vaginal dryness. More recently, physicians have realized that long-term use can reduce illness and death from heart disease and bone loss (osteoporosis). These potential benefits, however, are balanced to some extent by a possible increased risk of cancer, especially of the breast and uterus.

Indeed, it is largely fear of breast cancer, the most common cancer in women in the United States, that fuels the debate about hormone replacement. But in weighing the risks and benefits, we must recall that heart disease is the most prevalent cause of death for American women. In 1992 approximately 250,000 women died of coronary disease. Cancer ran a close second at 245,000 deaths for all types; the top three—lung, breast and colorectal cancer—account for 55,000, 43,000 and 29,000 deaths, respectively.

How much do we know about the impact of hormone replacement therapy on heart disease, osteoporosis and cancer? A number of studies have suggested that the use of estrogen for several years decreases risk of heart disease by up to 50 percent—a critical finding in view of the prevalence of coronary disease among women in this country. Long-term hormone therapy also appears to be valuable in preventing the bone fractures that stem from osteoporosis. Hip fractures, which afflict over 175,000 women in the United States every year, can destroy vitality, lower the quality of life and lead to death. Sustained use of estrogen appears to reduce hip fractures by 30 to 40 percent; fractures at other sites seem to decrease as well. Furthermore, preliminary evidence hints that the therapy may offer some degree of protection against Alzheimer's disease. Its usefulness in preserving function of the genitourinary tract and in preventing tissue atrophy is well documented.

Most research shows that the greatest benefits of estrogen replacement come with continuous use that begins shortly after menopause. The bone-protecting effects, in particular, diminish rapidly within a few years of stopping medication. Unfortunately, this need for long-term use raises the fear that estrogen replacement might also be linked to the development of two hormonally related cancers, uterine and breast cancer.

Unequivocal evidence suggests that estrogen therapy increases the risk of uterine cancer by up to six-fold over that seen in women who do not take estrogens. Uterine cancer, however, is usually diagnosed early, and thus many deaths from the disease can be prevented (about 6,000 women die from this type of cancer every year). Even more important, the addition of another hormone, a progestin, markedly lessens the possibility of uterine cancer. This finding has led to the frequent prescription of estrogen and progestin together as a means of trying to maintain the cardiac and bone benefits of estrogen without increasing the likelihood of uterine cancer.

What about the effects of hormone replacement on breast cancer? That breast cancer is in part hormonally mediated is known from extensive epidemiologic studies. But the connection between breast cancer and hormonal therapy is not clear. Several dozen studies of various types have yielded mixed results. In aggregate, they suggest that less than five years of estrogen therapy has no impact on breast cancer. Some studies, however, show that the risk of breast cancer increases by 15 to 40 percent after longer durations of estrogen replacement, with or without progestin. Thus, long-term replacement, which has optimal effects on heart disease and osteoporosis, may well be linked to a small increase in the incidence of breast cancer.

A little known finding is that hormone replacement therapy appears to offer some protection against another deadly malignancy, colon cancer.

Several studies now indicate that women taking hormone replacement therapy have half the chance of dying from colon cancer when compared with those who are not taking hormones.

Given the uncertainty about the exact impact of this therapy, the National Institutes of Health has launched a 15-year, nationwide clinical trial involving postmenopausal women. Called the Women's Health Initiative, it will evaluate the total health effects of hormone replacement therapy. Women who have had a hysterectomy and therefore have no risk of uterine cancer will be randomly assigned to daily estrogen or a placebo; those with an intact uterus will be assigned to daily estrogen plus progestin or will be given a placebo. This trial will focus on heart disease and osteoporotic fractures, but information about breast and colon cancer may also emerge, with the earliest findings expected at the beginning of the next century.

In the meantime, women must be guided by their own concerns and personal health histories, as well as by the relative impact of heart disease, osteoporosis and cancer of the breast, colon and uterus on women's health in general. Doctors should advise women who choose not to take hormones of other ways to minimize heart disease and osteoporosis. Alternative approaches to protecting the heart include not smoking; following a regular exercise program; taking aspirin; and getting treatment for high blood pressure, high cholesterol and diabetes. Women can minimize bone loss through exercise, calcium intake and the judicious use of antiosteoporotic medications. For many women, however, the potential benefits of hormone therapy on heart, bone, colon and quality of life will outweigh the risk of breast cancer.

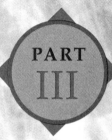

# TOWARD EARLIER DETECTION

New technology promises not only to detect cancers earlier and more accurately but also to catch tumors in their precancerous state, when the disease still might be prevented outright. The same basic instruments should help physicians to distinguish patients who need minimal treatment from those who need the most aggressive interventions.

# Advances in Cancer Detection

*Tests to look for the presence of a tumor before any symptoms
appear may save more lives than new drug therapies*

• • •

David Sidransky

A woman walks into a doctor's office after having felt a lump in her breast. The doctor feels the mass and an all too familiar story ensues. A biopsy confirms a diagnosis of breast cancer. Surgery and perhaps radiation or chemotherapy are prescribed. This scenario frequently results in a poor outcome simply because the tumor is found only after symptoms appear.

Many people have come to know the early symptoms of cancer through the American Cancer Society's self-screening guidelines. But by the time symptoms occur—usually pain or bleeding from an organ or a noticeable mass or lump—many tumors have already grown quite large. Despite aggressive surgery to remove the tumor, many advanced cancers recur or have metastasized and may end a patient's life. Tumors that are small, in contrast, are less apt to have spread and more likely to be eradicated.

A recent revolution in molecular biology and our understanding of cancer genetics has contributed to the development of a series of promising tests both for assessing one's risk of getting cancer and for discovering tumors while they are small enough for surgery to be effective. Still other assays may determine the best form of chemotherapy for a given patient or the likelihood that a cancer will recur after surgery. Instead of using invasive probes, the tests can be conducted with a small sample of urine or a pinprick of blood. Despite the long-standing emphasis on new treatments for cancer, such as gene therapy, many of us believe that early detection and improved monitoring will save the most lives in the years to come, by making it possible for existing therapies to be applied at a time when they can be most effective.

## A Genetic Legacy

As is true of many other diseases, the tendency to contract a particular cancer can be inherited. Mutations in specific genes passed from parent to child determine susceptibility to a number of breast and colon cancers, melanomas and other, rarer tumor types. Simple blood tests are now under development to hunt for DNA mutations in the two known breast cancer susceptibility genes (*BRCA1* and *BRCA2*). The tests will help assess risk for early-onset breast cancer. If a woman carries this mutation she faces a high likelihood, though not a certainty, of developing breast cancer, usually before her 40th birthday. (Men are confronted with a degree of increased risk for breast and possibly prostate cancer.)

Conversely, if a woman is not a carrier of the mutation, her risk of breast cancer may be no higher than that for the general population (about one in eight women will get the disease during their lifetime). The new tests will allow physicians to monitor closely members of genetically susceptible families (see Figure 6.1). Mammography and other conventional surveillance may then detect tumors that are still tiny. But because only a small proportion of cancers are thought to be inherited—about 10 percent of all cases—these tests may be of value only in high-risk families. Besides breast cancer, other genetic tests for cancer susceptibility will become available—for colon cancer, for example.

The ability to determine a person's risk for cancer decades in advance of the possible onset of the disease itself raises an array of social and even psychological issues. Legislators have already begun to pass laws to prevent discrimination by insurers against carriers of gene mutations. Knowledge of one's genetic legacy can also become a terrible psychological burden that must be borne by entire families.

Even members of a family who are not carriers of the mutation must cope with associated guilt feelings (see the box "Is Genetic Testing Premature?").

In addition to the social problems, a number of technical hurdles must be overcome before testing becomes widely practiced. Despite significant advances in genetic techniques, the ability to devise reliable tests that will detect cancer-related mutations remains a challenge. Cases will be missed if a test does not find all mutations that may lead to malignancies. Besides being accurate, any test must help improve survival rates—a goal that has yet to be decisively demonstrated. Some critics of susceptibility tests assert that intensive monitoring following a positive test—a routine schedule of mammograms, for example—may fail to turn up tumors early enough to improve a patient's chances of recovery. Still, evidence from studies of families that carry a high risk of contracting cancer of the colon suggests that close surveillance, medication with chemical agents that prevent cancer and, in some cases, removal of the colon can dramatically reduce mortality.

The preemptive option of excising an organ such as the colon or breast may not be fully preventive. For example, after a mastectomy, some cancerous breast tissue may be left behind, although the risk

Figure 6.1 CANCER SUSCEPTIBILITY can sometimes be tracked by testing for genetic mutations. Scientists at the Johns Hopkins University School of Medicine are searching through the genes of the Lueder family of Omaha, Neb., for a mutation linked to a colon cancer syndrome, which is also implicated in cancers of the urinary tract. The genes involved reside in sections of three chromosomes (*gray in diagram*).

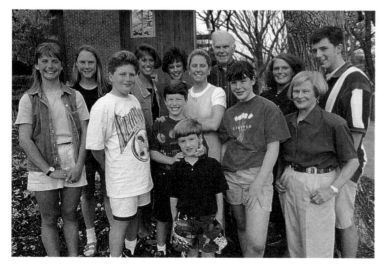

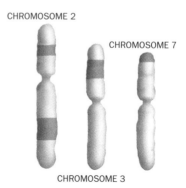

CHROMOSOME 2

CHROMOSOME 7

CHROMOSOME 3

# Some Family Cancer Syndromes

| SYNDROME[1] | CANCER | GENE | DNA TESTING COST[2] |
|---|---|---|---|
| Familial melanoma | Melanoma, pancreatic | *MTS1/p16* (tumor suppressor gene) | $400–$600 |
| Hereditary breast or ovarian cancer | Breast, ovarian, others | *BRCA1* (tumor suppressor gene) | $400–$2,000 |
| Hereditary breast cancer | Breast, others | *BRCA2* (tumor suppressor gene) | $400–$2,000 |
| Hereditary non-polyposis colon cancer | Colon, uterine, others | *MSH2, MLH1, PMS1, PMS2* (tumor suppressor genes) | $400–$2,000 |
| Li-Fraumeni syndrome | Brain, sarcomas, others | *p53* (tumor suppressing gene) | $500–$700 |
| Multiple endocrine neoplasia | Medullary thyroid, others | *RET* (oncogene) | $350–500 |

[1] Syndromes may encompass several types of cancer.
[2] Costs depend on amount of testing needed.

that a tumor may still arise is diminished. The inherent shortfalls of testing for susceptibility highlight the need to develop better strategies for early detection—the discovery of tumors when they are quite small or just beginning to become malignant. Improved detection should help not only families with inherited susceptibility but also the population at large.

Whether genetic changes are inherited, as in family cancer syndromes, or entirely acquired in the course of a lifetime, cancer ultimately results from alterations to DNA, our genetic code. To become aggressively malignant—proliferating uncontrollably, infiltrating other tissues and metastasizing—cells must sustain damage to a number of cancer-related genes (see Chapter 1, "How Cancer Arises"). From our broadening understanding of the disease, we now know that small clusters of precancerous cells (still considered benign but on their way to developing into cancer) and early cancers frequently harbor detectable genetic changes—a finding that opens new approaches to testing.

## Molecular Probes

Existing cytological analyses—examination under a microscope of cells from a Pap smear, for instance—are often insufficient for identifying a small number of abnormal cells by size and shape alone. DNA analysis, however, can detect tiny groups of mutated cells that are shed from a newly cancerous organ into bodily fluids—ranging from urine to sputum or even fluids excreted from the nipples. A technique called polymerase chain reaction (PCR) permits more than a million copies to be made from a single strand of DNA present in a precancerous or cancerous cell. This molecular reproduction biotechnology allows testing to be conducted on clinical samples as small as a single drop of fluid.

The DNA copied through PCR can then be hybridized: the two strands of the familiar DNA "ladder" are separated, then exposed to genetic probes consisting of a single strand of DNA that contains a specific mutation commonly found in a cancer cell. Any DNA in a sample of fluid that has

# Is Genetic Testing Premature?

The ability to pinpoint inherited genetic mutations that predispose a person to cancer has generated a firestorm of controversy within the medical establishment. During the 1980s, researchers identified the first marker for cancer susceptibility—a genetic mutation that causes retinoblastoma, a malignancy of the eye. But it was the discovery during the mid-1990s of genes involved in breast cancer—and the subsequent development of tests that could assess susceptibility to the disease—that brought the issue to the forefront of public debate. The importance of finding the breast cancer genes goes beyond that illness alone, given that the genes can predispose both men or women to a variety of other malignancies, from ovarian to, possibly, prostate cancer.

The dilemma for both ethicists and physicians revolves around the still cloudy meaning of test results. If a test affirms the presence of a genetic mutation, a woman with a family history of breast cancer faces an 85 percent risk—not a certainty—of contracting the disease. But the risks are not yet known for a woman with the mutation who does not have any relatives who have had the disease.

Even with test results in hand, a woman will face difficult decisions about what to do with this knowledge. A negative test for an inherited genetic defect may give her an unwarranted sense of complacency, because about 85 percent of cancers are not inherited, and she remains at risk for acquiring the noninheritable type. She may also have inherited mutations that lead to the disease that have yet to be identified by researchers.

A positive test also provides less than clear-cut options. Increased monitoring may prove inadequate: mammography can overlook a tumor. And preventive removal of both breasts provides no guarantee that the tissue left after surgery will remain free of cancer.

Critics of testing worry about abuse of this information by insurers and employers. A number of states have already passed laws to prevent health insurance providers from using genetic tests to discriminate against patients. Moreover, federal legislation that would outlaw such discrimination has been working its way through Congress. Until some of these issues can be resolved, the National Breast Cancer Coalition, the American Society of Human Genetics and the National Advisory Council for Human Genome Research have recommended that testing be conducted only as part of an ongoing research effort.

Nevertheless, the rush to test outside the research environment has started. One clinic—Genetics & I.V.F. Institute in Fairfax, Va.—offers a test for a mutation found in Ashkenazi Jewish women. Two companies—Myriad Genetics and OncorMed—have developed more comprehensive tests that look for a broader range of mutations in both the known breast cancer genes, *BRCA1* and *BRCA2*. These tests are expected to come into routine clinical use in a few years.

---

the same mutation binds to the probe, which can be tagged with a fluorescent dye or radioactive material (see the box "Diagnosing Hubert H. Humphrey 27 Years Later").

Much of the work on DNA analysis for cancer detection has been carried out at my laboratory at the Johns Hopkins University School of Medicine. Using these molecular-based methods, my colleagues and I have found telltale cancer gene mutations—in the sputum for lung cancer, in the urine for bladder cancer and in the stool for colon cancer. Several years ago our team demonstrated that mutations could be detected in a cancer gene called *ras* by looking in the stool of patients with polyps—growths in the colon that are precursors of colon cancer. The mutations also appeared in patients in whom colon cancer had already developed.

These results have led to larger trials to determine if identification of *ras* gene mutations in the stool may become a general screening strategy. Such a test may find polyps before they show up through colonoscopy (inspection of the colon with a colonoscope). The simple removal of a polyp greatly diminishes a patient's chances of acquiring cancer.

A test for *ras* mutations may become routine in medical laboratories within a few years. But using this type of genetic assay may prove too time-consuming and costly when searching for the mul-

The medical establishment's consensus in opposing clinical testing outside a research study has already begun to weaken. In the May issue of the *Journal of Clinical Oncology*, the American Society of Clinical Oncology broke ranks with other groups by recommending that testing be permitted for anyone with a family history of breast cancer. Advocates of testing believe that ignoring available genetic information can place a patient at risk. The ambiguities and anxieties that accompany testing, they contend, can be addressed through proper counseling. David Sidransky takes that view. Sidransky, who is affiliated with the Johns Hopkins University School of Medicine and who advises OncorMed, points out that even without genetic susceptibility testing, aggressive surveillance of patients at high risk for colon cancer has led to a dramatic decrease in mortality.

Sidransky suggests that women with a breast cancer gene mutation might enter an intensive surveillance regimen and might be eligible for clinical trials of new types of chemoprevention compounds. Knowing that one harbors a mutation may cause stress to the patient and her family, Sidransky acknowledges. "These issues don't compare, though, to getting metastatic breast cancer and dying from the disease," he adds.

Other observers lack Sidransky's certitude. Francis S. Collins, who heads the National Center for Human Genome Research, collaborated on a response to the policy statement in the *Journal of Clinical Oncology*. "We are concerned," the statement noted, "that the ability to test for hereditary susceptibility will precede the ability to inform individuals of their best medical choices, to provide counseling and education that will help individuals and families make decisions that affect quality of life, and to protect families from various forms of discrimination." Collins submitted the reply on behalf of the National Action Plan on Breast Cancer, a public-private partnership.

Collins points to the National Cancer Institute's recently established National Cancer Genetics Network as a means for patients to enroll in a research study and thus learn of their genetic status while receiving counseling. The network will give patients and their physicians a mechanism for coping with the troubling knowledge of being a carrier of a mutated gene.

— Gary Stix

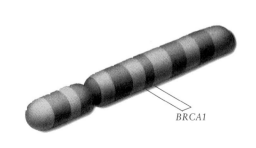

BRCA1

tiple mutations that can be found in some genes. A separate DNA probe must ferret out each mutation. An alternative approach to spotting malignancies employs small pieces of repetitive DNA called microsatellites. Because these repeating units contain no useful information for a cell, they are sometimes referred to as junk DNA. Still, microsatellites hold a wealth of information for the cancer diagnostician and also for forensics specialists who employ them as one of the DNA fingerprinting methods that received much attention during the O. J. Simpson trial.

Spread throughout the DNA in every chromosome, microsatellites have begun to prove their worth in cancer diagnosis. The absence of a cluster of these repetitive units indicates deletion of a region of a chromosome. And a change in size of the microsatellites also confirms a genetic alteration.

In one small trial, we at Johns Hopkins tested patients who showed symptoms of bladder cancer for the presence of abnormal microsatellites in their urine. We discovered microsatellite changes by comparing the DNA in the urine to that in blood. The bladder casts off cancer cells into the urine but leaves blood untainted. The blood acts as a control sample against which the urine can be tested.

In 19 of 20 of these patients, we found changes in microsatellite DNA pointing to the absence of an

## Diagnosing Hubert H. Humphrey 27 Years Later

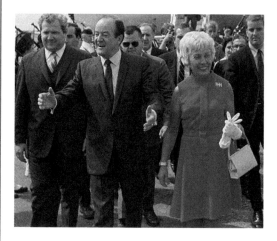

Excerpt from a letter from Muriel Humphrey Brown, Hubert H. Humphrey's widow, giving permission to the Johns Hopkins University School of Medicine to use her late husband's medical samples. Her decision, she says, would have concurred with his wishes.

*"This is what Hubert would have wanted; this is what kept him going, I believe, and this is why we wanted his records to be preserved for future use.*

*Hubert and I had a philosophy that saw us through many hard times. It was 'Everything happens for the best.' Often, it takes a long time to know why. Through many years of grief and anger, I couldn't relate our philosophy to his suffering and death. Perhaps now I have the answer."*

The power of the new molecular diagnostic tools became apparent in 1994, when our team of researchers at the Johns Hopkins University School of Medicine diagnosed Hubert H. Humphrey's bladder cancer from a 27-year-old urine sample. Humphrey had a classic case, one that underscores the need for early detection

In 1967, when he held the office of vice president, he found blood in his urine. His doctors performed tests to look for abnormal cells. they could not, however, make a definitive finding of cancer, and so aggressive treatment was delayed. A few years later the correct diagnosis was made, and in 1976 Humphrey underwent radiation therapy and radical surgery. He eventually died when the disease recurred.

In the experiment (see diagram), the researchers—Ralph H. Hruban, Peter van der Riet, Yener S. Erozan and I—were given permission by Humphrey's widow, Muriel Humphrey Brown, to work with urine samples that were taken in 1967 and a sample of the tumor removed years later.

Today we know that certain mutations in the *p53* gene constitute signs of bladder cancer. But we wanted to know if such a mutation had been detectable in 1967 in Humphrey's urine. To find out, we first confirmed that the tumor carried a *p53* mutation (bottom of diagram). We extracted and made copies of DNA and then sequenced (identified each nucleotide, or DNA building block) in a part of the *p53* gene. Sequencing revealed a point mutation: one nucleotide (adenine) had been replaced by another (thymine). We then synthesized a probe consisting of a single strand of DNA that would recognize, or pair with, DNA carrying the same mutation. A radioactive label was attached to the DNA strands to keep track of the probe.

entire region of a chromosome. The same alterations were then documented in biopsies of tumors taken from the patients. In patients without cancer, we did not find abnormal microsatellites. Although the test missed one patient, the 95 percent detection rate compares favorably with the record of less sophisticated diagnostic techniques, such as the Pap smears that detect cervical cancer.

The simplicity and low cost of microsatellite testing give it an advantage over detection of specific genetic mutations such as *ras*. In fact, the whole technique can be automated: a technician will need only a drop of urine and blood. At the press of a button, a machine that performs PCR will make copies of DNA from a urine sample to identify a microsatellite pattern that confirms the presence of

Separately, we made copies of the DNA from the *p53* gene in the urine sample (top of diagram) using a technique called the polymerase chain reaction (PCR). We then inserted the DNA into bacteria, which grew into colonies that were placed on a nylon membrane. In the colonies, the DNA strands were separated (so that they would be amenable to pairing with the right probe). When the probes were placed on the membrane (far right), they paired with DNA in the bacteria that contained the mutation—indicating that the mutation had indeed been present in Humphrey's urine as early as 1967.

Similar methods have been used to devise the tests that are coming into clinical use for cancer detection. Urine or blood can be subjected to a probe that pinpoints a known mutation for cancer.

Humphrey's case highlights the potential of new molecular approaches to make positive diagnoses when other techniques show equivocal results. An earlier diagnosis could have resulted in lifesaving surgery years earlier and might have changed the course of political history. Humphrey might have even had second thoughts about his decision to run for president against Richard M. Nixon in the 1968 campaign.

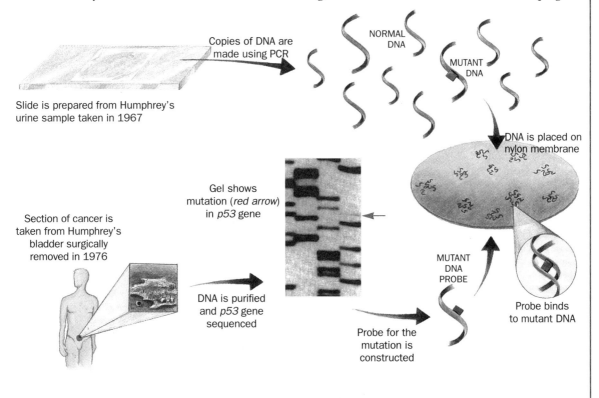

Copies of DNA are made using PCR

Slide is prepared from Humphrey's urine sample taken in 1967

NORMAL DNA

MUTANT DNA

DNA is placed on nylon membrane

Gel shows mutation (*red arrow*) in *p53* gene

Section of cancer is taken from Humphrey's bladder surgically removed in 1976

DNA is purified and *p53* gene sequenced

MUTANT DNA PROBE

Probe binds to mutant DNA

Probe for the mutation is constructed

bladder cancer. Larger trials have now begun to validate our preliminary results. It still remains to be determined whether this approach will work for all cancers.

Other strategies for early detection have focused on monitoring the levels of proteins that are either the product of a mutated gene or are present as a consequence of the unique biochemistry of a par-ticular cancer. An example is circulating PSA (prostate-specific antigen) in the blood of patients with prostate cancer (see "Current Controversy: Does Screening for Prostate Cancer Make Sense?," following Chapter 7). PSA testing has an established role in monitoring the progress of prostate cancer patients: high levels of the protein signify a recurrence of a malignancy. But the test may ultimately prove to be a reliable tool for early detection. Many doctors have already begun to use it routinely for detecting prostate tumors.

### Enzyme Markers

A simple protein test that has shown promise for both detection and monitoring looks for an enzyme, called telomerase, that is active when cancer arises. The enzyme affects telomeres—the segments at the ends of chromosomes that grow progressively shorter each time a cell divides. When telomeres shorten to a certain length, they instruct the cell to self-destruct, providing a mechanism to rid the body of aging cells. In most normal cells, telomerase is absent, but in cancer, it is active and blocks telomere shortening. Consequently, the malignant cells do not die.

Because the enzyme is rarely present in normal cells, it can serve as a marker to signal the early presence of cancer cells. In theory, telomerase screening holds the prospect of providing a general strategy for detection of cancer in bodily fluids and tissue. Geron, a company based in Menlo Park, Calif., has begun development of a test for telomerase activity based on research carried out by Jerry W. Shay of the University of Texas Southwestern Medical Center and Carol Greider of Cold Spring Harbor Laboratory.

Research on protein tests actually predates the advent of testing for genetic markers. Many of the tests, however, have failed to live up to expectations because they produce too many false results. For this reason, recent efforts have tended to shift toward investigations into genetic pathways.

Besides early detection, clinicians must ascertain how readily a particular tumor will grow or spread. This assessment—a process called staging—becomes a critical component in determining what additional treatment the patient will receive after surgery—either radiation or chemotherapy. In staging, doctors examine pieces of tissue to make sure that all the tumor has been removed. But tumor cells also may drain into nearby lymph nodes. The number of nodes involved after tumor removal is important in establishing the prognosis.

Physicians have long been aware that the standard approach to staging—identifying abnormal cells under the light microscope—often fails to turn up very small populations of cancer cells.

Recently our team at Johns Hopkins has applied molecular technology to detect hidden malignant cells in patients with cancer of the voice box and other head and neck cancers. Despite aggressive surgery, these tumors often recur in the same area. In a pilot study, we examined patients whose tumors were known to harbor mutations in a gene known as *p53*. The *p53* gene is a tumor suppressor gene that normally inhibits unchecked cell growth; when it becomes inactive, cells often grow cancerous.

We developed molecular probes for *p53* that we used to test the lymph nodes and nearby tissue remaining after the tumor's ostensibly complete removal. In more than half the cases, there was at least one area surrounding the tumor that, though negative under the light microscope, contained cells with the same *p53* mutations as the tumor. These cancer cells had spread into tissue surrounding the lymph nodes and were left behind after the surgery was done.

In patients with a positive test, cancer often recurred—and the site of its reappearance was frequently the same area where we had originally detected the presence of malignant cells. In contrast, those patients who tested negative after surgery have yet to experience another episode of the disease. Other investigators have also identified these mutations in the lymph nodes of patients with colon cancer.

Such molecular markers as the *p53* gene may also help evaluate how patients will respond to various forms of chemotherapy. The normal function of *p53* is to sense genetic damage and then to lead a cell to its own death—the progression of cellular events called apoptosis. Many types of chemotherapy work by causing genetic damage to cells, which would usually trigger the *p53* gene to initiate apoptosis. But tumors in which the *p53* gene has been deleted or rendered inactive may not respond to certain types of conventional chemotherapy. In breast cancer, alternative chemotherapies, such as taxol, which may not rely on *p53* to bring about apoptosis, are now being considered in patients with *p53* mutant tumors.

For genetic detection and monitoring to fulfill its potential, merely sensing the presence of a mutated gene will not be enough. It will be necessary to pinpoint the location of a tiny clump of malignant cells so they can be excised. Improvements in imaging techniques—magnetic resonance imaging or computed tomography—will help detect such lesions. These studies can be augmented by "biological" imaging—the ingestion of low-level radioactive compounds or the use of fluorescent techniques whose radiation signals a tumor's whereabouts.

Despite the benefits of molecular detection, most of the studies mentioned in this chapter are still quite preliminary and await final validation in large clinical trials. Still, I remain quite optimistic that within five years, molecular detection—and subsequent strategies for staging and tailoring treatment approaches—will be part of a routine physical examination for most people in the United States.

There will probably never be a single test that can detect every kind of tumor. Each cancer has its own molecular signature and so will require its own test. Even so, the genetic changes that lead to cancer may also become the disease's ultimate weak point. We can envision the time when a minuscule sample of blood, tissue or various bodily fluids will reveal the presence of a new or metastatic tumor—be it of the lung, breast, colon or another organ—in time to eradicate it. The sensitivity of these test may change our fundamental conception of cancer. Rather than becoming a frightful diagnosis linked to an inevitable tragedy, early-stage tumors will be caught and cured.

# Advances in Tumor Imaging

*New tools yield a three-dimensional view inside the body
and automated advice on interpreting the anatomical landscape.*

• • •

Maryellen L. Giger and Charles A. Pelizzari

During the past five years, improvements in medical imaging technology have enabled radiologists to make pictures of the human body with unprecedented resolution and clarity. Meanwhile the rapid increase in available computer power has encouraged researchers to develop highly sophisticated techniques for displaying and analyzing those images.

Although radiologists' attention has focused on such advanced techniques as positron-emission tomography (PET) and magnetic resonance imaging (MRI), both of which can map physiological functions as they take place, the needs of cancer specialists are somewhat different. They require tools that can tease out the subtle differences between cancerous tissue and normal body cells. As yet, however, no imaging technique can identify tumors unambiguously—imaging can only guide more direct explorations, usually by surgery and examination of tissue samples.

Two new technologies for cancer detection and therapy are three-dimensional multimodality display and computer-aided diagnosis. The display technique employs scientific visualization methods similar to those used in the geosciences or astronomy to fuse information from several imaging tools into a single coherent picture. In the second technique, software incorporating artificial intelligence and machine-vision algorithms can scan mammograms and chest x-rays for telltale signs of cancer. Both methods have adapted software and hardware originally developed for other purposes and turned it to oncological ends. Neither is currently in widespread use, but both appear to be making their way out of the laboratory.

A complete and effective display of the relevant image data for a case can aid physicians in making a precise diagnosis and in designing the best treatment, whether by surgery, radiation or chemotherapy. Current x-ray computed tomographic (CT) scanners, for example, can quickly produce detailed 3-D images of anatomical features.

## Three-Dimensional Imaging

In a CT scan, bones appear bright and distinct, but soft tissue such as muscle, blood vessels and tumors frequently appears in almost identical

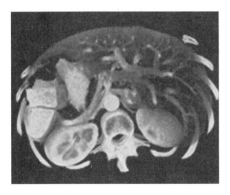 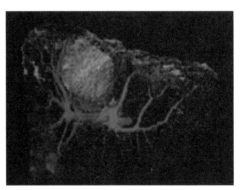 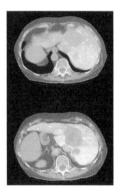

**Figure 7.1 COMPUTED TOMOGRAPHIC SCAN** data can be viewed in many different ways to aid physicians in identifying tumors and planning treatment. The image at the left shows a normal liver and most of the torso, as seen from above. A more specialized image (*center*) focuses on a cancerous liver. Normal liver tissue has been rendered mostly transparent, tumor tissue has been colored yellow and hepatic arteries red. Such a display is far more useful than conventional CT slices (*right*).

shades of gray (see Figure 7.1). Radiologists can inject contrast agents containing such heavy atoms as iodine to make blood vessels stand out, but modern digital processing is even more valuable for enhancing images. In the past, physicians had to rely on examination of multiple two-dimensional slices rather than 3-D views of an entire data set because of the large volume of data involved. Now high-performance computers and dedicated graphics hardware can display detailed 3-D medical data easily, rotating, magnifying or panning images in as little as a few seconds.

The computer can also add color to images so that the varying shades of x-ray absorption corresponding to different kinds of tissue are immediately distinguishable; the resulting 3-D visualizations aid in understanding the structures of tumors and their relation to the surrounding, normal anatomy. Doctors can readily determine, for example, whether a tumor has infiltrated vital tissues or grown around blood vessels in ways that could complicate its surgical removal.

Other advanced medical imaging methods, including MRI, PET and single-photon-emission computed tomography (SPECT), can produce 3-D images of physiological functions such as blood flow, oxygen consumption or glucose metabolism. MRI, for example, is sensitive to differences in chemical composition and fluid content, and so tumors (whose consistency differs from that of normal tissue) often present a more dramatic, readily comprehensible appearance in these images than in CT. Intact bones contain relatively little fluid and

thus appear dark in MRI. PET and SPECT, on the other hand, produce only images of biological functions—they do not show either bones or organs directly. Because PET and SPECT also have limited resolution, they cannot show as much detail as CT or MRI; consequently, the increase in functional information about blood flow and cell metabolism—which can help a doctor understand a tumor's behavior or its response to therapy—is counterbalanced by the loss of precise locational information.

Each of these imaging technologies is currently in use on its own. And although information from a single kind of scan can help assess the location and spread of tumors and identify nearby critical anatomical structures such as organs, nerves and vasculature, the information each method provides often complements that yielded by the others. A view based on several different imaging techniques can be particularly useful. Radiologists may merge PET or SPECT data with an MRI or CT image so they can determine more exactly the metabolic activity of various parts of malignant and normal tissue.

Researchers have recently developed methods for fusing images more precisely by transforming them so that they all have a common scale and spatial reference frame. These image-registration techniques are especially important for smaller tumors. Images can also be overlaid with information from other sources such as radiation-dose calculations. Specialists can then see precisely what regions will be affected by a course of therapy (see Figure 7.2).

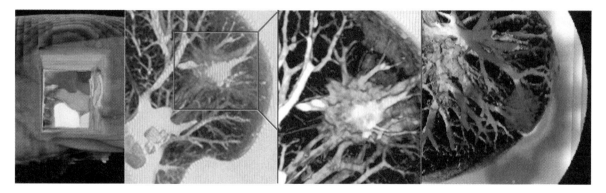

Figure 7.2  3-D RECONSTRUCTIONS can help physicians plan surgery or radiation treatment. Specialized display software can hide irrelevant or obscuring features (as in the view of the prostate at the left). Radiologists magnify areas of interest (such as a lung tumor in the two middle views) and merge CT scan data with other information, as in the image at right. The colored contours indicate the radiation dose from a particular configuration of beams; blue and green represent the lowest exposure; red is the highest.

Those who have used these tools are convinced that they improve patient care, but rigorous trials to validate this impression have yet to be designed.

## Computer-Aided Diagnosis

In addition to techniques that let physicians see more clearly inside the body, researchers are also developing tools that could help them interpret the images they see. Computer-aided diagnostic tools do not make a definitive decision about the implications of a mammogram or other test; instead they offer an automated "second opinion." We have found that computers analyze images in different ways than people do—the kinds of patterns that machine-vision algorithms can easily identify are not the same as the patterns caught by the human visual system. As a result, computers can complement the radiologist's eye. And the availability of high-quality digitizers and fast computers makes it possible to process medical images in minutes.

Most of the effort expended so far in this area has been on detecting and characterizing abnormalities in digitized mammograms and chest radiographs. Computer-aided diagnostic methods may direct radiologists' attention to suspect regions and so prevent errors of oversight. Such systems are only now progressing beyond the early stages, and many screening cases will need to be analyzed before a final assessment can be made, but initial studies suggest impressive effectiveness.

Although mammography is currently the best method for the detection of breast cancer, some tumors are still difficult to detect. Between 10 and 30 percent of women who undergo mammography and turn out to have breast cancer initially register negative results. These false negatives may occur because of lesions that are intrinsically difficult to detect, poor image quality, eye fatigue or simple oversight. The interpretation of mammograms is a repetitive task that requires attention to minute detail. Out of every 1,000 sets of mammograms taken for screening purposes, only about five will actually contain images of cancerous lesions. When two radiologists read the same film, the sensitivity for detection of lesions can increase by 15 percent. This situation suggests that the task of evaluating mammograms may lend itself well to automated computer analysis, to take at least some of the burden from the radiologist. An intelligent workstation would serve as a second reader (like a spell-checker for computerized texts), leaving the final decision regarding the likelihood of the presence of cancer to the radiologist.

At the Kurt Rossmann Laboratories of the University of Chicago's department of radiology, we have been developing such a workstation, which employs various algorithms in computer vision and artificial intelligence to detect breast cancers. We tested the detection software on archived mammograms that had already been manually examined and found that it pointed out 90 percent of the lesions while raising only two false positive queries per mammogram. (A false positive is an area that the program rates as suspicious but that the radiologist ultimately decides does not

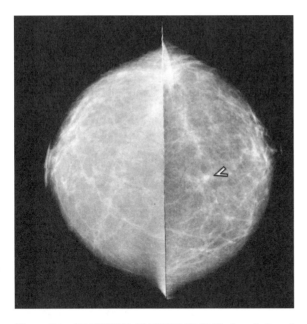

**Figure 7.3   ARCHIVED MAMMOGRAMS show left and right breasts of a woman who was later discovered to have breast cancer. Computerized reexamination of these earlier films pointed out a lesion (*arrow*) that had been missed by a radiologist. Such image-analysis software could improve the effectiveness of mammographic screening.**

reading, but when a patient showed up with a growth at her next mammographic exam, a second look disclosed signs of cancer on the original film. The computer detected approximately half the lesions, while generating an average of two false positives per image. Had the software been in place at the time, the computer might have helped radiologists find half the cancers that they initially overlooked, resulting in earlier and simpler treatment as well as improving the chances for a cure.

Since November 1994 our intelligent workstation has been analyzing screening mammograms (those taken to check for possible malignancies rather than to monitor ongoing conditions) as they are taken. For each exam, a laser scanner digitizes two images of each breast and converts the film's shades of gray to arrays of numbers in the computer (see Figure 7.3). Image-processing techniques deemphasize background structures and enhance others, such as calcified regions, that may be of diagnostic importance. Feature-extraction software recognizes specific characteristics of individual image regions, classifying them by shape or contrast. Masses whose edges contain many sharp spicules, for example, indicate malignancy. The software can also merge characteristics of the image singled out by the radiologist with those extracted by the computer to aid in diagnosis. Further analysis employs explicit sets of rules about image characteristics and "neural network" software, applied to collections of both cancerous and normal images, to cull the list of suspicious regions and so reduce the number of false positive detections.

As these sophisticated imaging techniques and computer-aided diagnostic software enter more widespread clinical testing, some patients will benefit from them almost immediately. But the ultimate impact of the technology will not be seen for a decade or more.

represent a possible malignancy; radiology residents in training typically generate several false positives per image.) The program flagged 85 percent of clustered microcalcifications, a different kind of abnormality that can also signal cancerous conditions, including ductal carcinoma in situ (DCIS). The software generated only 0.6 false positive per image while searching for these tiny spots, which radiologists may sometimes overlook.

We also tested the software on a missed-lesion database. These mammograms, collected over several years, had been classed as tumor-free on first

# Current Controversy: Should Women in Their 40s Have Mammograms?

• • •

Gina Maranto

For at least four years now, breast cancer specialists have been heatedly arguing among themselves about whether women in their forties benefit from having routine mammograms. In 1993 the National Cancer Institute sparked the debate by proclaiming that women in this age group need not undergo such screening—a reversal of the NCI's previous position and the opposite of the American Cancer Society and of the American Medical Association recommendations.

Physicians, radiologists, statisticians and public health officials have made claims and counterclaims and—with sometimes startling emotion—have accused one another of misreading or misrepresenting data, of performing faulty analyses and of perpetuating myths that have dire consequences for women. Some specialists, as well as cancer societies, women's health advocates and manufacturers of mammography machines, have argued that mass screening saves lives; others on the clinical front lines and in policy-setting roles have contended that evidence from a number of randomized controlled trials does not support such a claim. Instead, they say, the data reveal that younger women whose breasts are scanned by x-rays die at the same rate as those whose breasts are manually examined by a physician on a regular basis.

Maybe the only true consensus to have emerged (at least among epidemiologists) from the protracted and politicized dispute is that it is not possible, given the current data, to prove beyond a statistical shadow of a doubt that mammography lowers the breast cancer death rate in women ages 40 to 49, although there are some who would challenge even this assertion. Given the disagreement, what's a woman to do?

For now, it appears that there are no unequivocal answers. Perhaps a woman's best bet is to educate herself about what mammography can and cannot do and then, with the aid of her physician, decide for herself what course to follow.

One key point to consider is that mammography, though apparently posing little (if any) risk of causing cancer, is not foolproof. By some estimates, 10 to 15 percent of women in any age group who walk away from a mammogram assured that they are free of cancer go on to acquire it within a year. In some cases, the disease stems from rapidly growing malignancies that emerged after screening; in others, from tumors that just failed to show up on the film. In addition, false negatives may result from a radiologist's lack of skill or experience, from too few readers (studies have shown that more cancers are caught by two independent readers than by a solo reader), from use of older equipment and because women in their forties often have dense breasts, which are harder to read clearly.

Mammography also results in a substantial number of false positive readings, and anyone undergoing the exam should brace herself for the possibility that her mammogram will fall among the 5 to 10 percent considered suspicious enough to warrant further investigation. And of these, the majority (between 60 and 93 percent) turn out to be associated with benign conditions.

But reaching a final determination may also require one or more biopsies under local or general anesthesia. Aside from the expense and time it takes, this process can also be physically taxing and anxiety-provoking. If the positive reading produces a diagnosis of ductal carcinoma in situ (DCIS)— and some 15 to 20 percent of "cancers" discovered by mammography fall into this category—the woman faces yet another decision for which medical science can offer only marginal assistance.

DCIS, which was virtually unknown before the development of mammography, does not proceed inevitably to invasive cancer. But with no way of telling when or whether the abnormal cells will escape from the constraining ducts and flare into deadly disease, most physicians recommend excising the affected area or, in some cases, the whole breast.

Yet even if a mammogram reveals an invasive malignancy that is still so small it cannot be felt, no one has been able to demonstrate indisputably that early detection reduces mortality. Which puts us back in the thick of the debate.

Daniel B. Kopans of Massachusetts General Hospital insists that faulty interpretations have muddied the picture and that when eight major studies of mammography are correctly analyzed, they show a clear benefit in terms of mortality reduction. Kopans has also written, in the volume *Important Advances in Oncology* (Philadelphia: J. B. Lippincott, 1995), that "screening for breast cancer is not, primarily, a public health issue, but a question for the woman who is interested in reducing her risk of dying from breast cancer."

Taking the opposite view, Cornelia J. Baines of the University of Toronto has made the case that catching cancers early, often before they can be felt, does not reduce the overall toll of the disease. Women trying to decide whether to undergo mammography, Baines wrote in the same volume, face an "uncomfortable choice. Will they choose to know they have breast cancer for the last 10 years of their life and to have a small tumor treated? Or will they choose to know they have breast cancer for the last five years of their life and to have a larger tumor treated?"

Despite reluctance to support broad-based screening programs, most experts in the field agree that women at high risk should receive regular mammograms. A strong factor raising a woman's risk is having a mother or sisters with breast cancer. Weaker factors include commencing menstruation before 12 years old; being childless or bearing one's first child after turning 30; or being obese.

Given that a woman's likelihood of acquiring breast cancer in her forties is less than 2 percent and that her chance of dying from it within a decade is even smaller, most women in this age group are unlikely to have to confront the disease. For those who do fall prey, the disquieting word from some specialists is that medicine can offer slim solace to those with the most aggressive form of the disease.

# Current Controversy: Does Screening for Prostate Cancer Make Sense?

• • •

Gerald E. Hanks and Peter T. Scardino

Since 1990 the reported number of new cases of prostate cancer has tripled, from fewer than 100,000 annually to an estimated 317,100 this year. The jump in incidence is largely the result of the introduction of tests, beginning in the late 1980s, that can signal the presence of previously undetectable cancer. By measuring the amount of a protein called prostate-specific antigen (PSA) in a male adult's blood, the tests may unmask a cancerous prostate five years or more before other symptoms arise (see the Figure "Small Percentage").

On its face, extending PSA testing to all men seems an obviously desirable goal. As a rule, the earlier someone's cancer is detected, the better the person's prospects for cure. And this cancer now takes a high toll: more than 40,000 men died of it in 1996, making it the second leading cause of cancer death (after lung cancer) and the sixth leading cause of death overall among American men. Prostate cancer is often characterized as a disease that older men die *with* rather than *of* (because it often progresses more slowly than other cancers do). Its incidence, mortality rate and mean age at diagnosis are in fact very similar to breast cancer statistics. Furthermore, once prostate cancer reaches an advanced stage, there is no effective therapy.

Yet many physicians, policymakers and patients are questioning the wisdom of widespread PSA screening. In addition to the billions of dollars required for universal screening and subsequent potential treatment, they are deterred by the fact that no one actually knows whether such testing would benefit the average man or reduce overall mortality for the population as a whole.

The favorable arguments are many. PSA is an effective screening tool: biopsies reveal cancer in about a third of men with elevated PSA levels. Screening clearly detects many tumors that would be missed by the traditional rectal examination, in which a physician feels the prostate. In addition, cancers detected by PSA screening are almost always larger and more aggressive than the indolent tumors found incidentally at autopsy in men who die of other causes.

PSA testing also often detects cancer at an early stage, when it is most likely to respond to treatment.

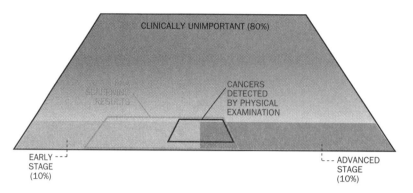

CLINICALLY UNIMPORTANT (80%)

PSA
SCREENING
RESULTS

CANCERS
DETECTED
BY PHYSICAL
EXAMINATION

EARLY
STAGE
(10%)

ADVANCED
STAGE
(10%)

SMALL PERCENTAGE of the estimated eight million American men who have cancerous cells in their prostate will be harmed by the disease. Of the cancers that could affect health, only about 6 percent are found by rectal examinations. Although critics of PSA screening worry that it will catch mostly insignificant or untreatable cancers, it appears to be detecting early, treatable ones instead (*green outline*).

Before PSA testing was introduced, two thirds of prostate cancers found had already spread beyond the prostate, making them essentially incurable. Most patients faced a choice between hormone therapy and removal of the testes, neither of which conferred more than a few years of survival. Today nearly two thirds of prostate cancers detected in screening programs and treated surgically are confined to the gland and can thus be eradicated by surgery or radiation.

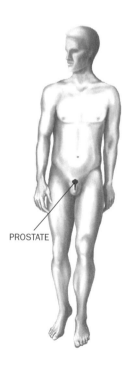

PROSTATE

For such reasons, both the American Cancer Society and the American Urological Association currently recommend that healthy men older than 50 years who have a life expectancy of at least 10 years undergo both rectal examination and PSA testing annually. Men at high risk for prostate cancer, including African-Americans (whose diet and average health care status appear to predispose them to the disease) and those with a family history of the disease, should begin testing at age 40.

At the same time, there is no unequivocal evidence that early detection through periodic screening with PSA measurements (or rectal examinations, for that matter) in fact reduces the chances of death from prostate cancer.

Some critics point to mortality figures as evidence that PSA testing does not save lives. They note that the enormous rise in early detection through PSA has not yielded a substantial change in death rates during the past decade. But this argument does not hold water. Because prostate cancer often progresses more slowly than other cancers, taking 10 years or more to become deadly, decreases in death rates would not be expected to show up for many years. If PSA screening does influence mortality, the effect probably will not be noticeable until after the turn of the century.

Other concerns about the value of PSA screening arise from the perhaps surprising fact that most growths of cancerous cells within the prostate do not lead to serious illness or death. A third of men over age 50 harbor some form of the cancer, but only between 6 and 10 percent will acquire the type likely to lead to death or disability. And only about 3 percent eventually die of it.

Most prostate tumors are tiny and consist of well-differentiated or moderately differentiated cells; they are unlikely to cause clinical disease within the remaining life expectancy of a man older than 70 years. A small proportion are large and contain highly irregular cells that metastasize early, killing patients within a few years of their spread to other parts of the body. Unfortunately for simple medical decision making, most malignancies detected today, especially by means of PSA tests, fall into an intermediate range whose variable natural history makes it difficult to distinguish those likely to progress rapidly from those that can safely be left alone.

Computer models of the value of early detection and treatment suggest that screening millions of men may offer little overall benefit to society in terms of either improved health or allocation of scarce medical resources. Critics worry about unnecessary costs and distress to patients. The two thirds of men who undergo biopsy as a result of elevated PSA only to learn that they have no apparent cancer are exposed to unwarranted stress and anxiety as well as some risk of infection and bleeding. To these negatives must be added the hazards of treatment (which can include urinary incontinence and impotence) for a further minority whose cancer would otherwise have remained undetected for the rest of their lives. The widespread use of PSA testing to screen men with no symptoms of prostate cancer, then, could mean that many tumors that would previously have had no effect on people's lives will now be detected and treated at substantial costs in dollars and in suffering. Only time will tell whether the count of significant yet treatable cancers uncovered—and the resulting survival benefits—outweighs these costs.

Assuming that a prostate cancer, once detected, is both dangerous and still potentially curable, there remains considerable controversy about how to treat it. The three best understood alternatives are "watchful waiting," external irradiation and surgical prostatectomy. The choice of treatment for any given case is a divisive issue for both physician and patient. Each has its pros and cons, and there is no consensus on which is best.

Radical prostatectomy has been used to treat prostate cancer since 1903. Since 1984 the number of operations performed each year has increased more than sixfold, with an estimated 160,000 done in 1995. Its major advantage is that if the disease is truly localized, cancerous cells can be removed completely, effectively curing the patient in as many as 70 percent of cases. More than four out of five patients who have no detectable PSA five years after surgery never show signs of recurrence.

The immediate price a patient pays for this effectiveness is a major operation with a stay in the hospital and an extended recovery. Longer-term side effects may include several months of urinary stress incontinence (with a chance of permanent incontinence between 3 and 5 percent) and six months to a year of erectile impotence (with a chance of permanent loss between 30 and 50 percent). The rate at which function returns (if it does) depends on the patient's age, previous state of sexual function and the extent of the operation to remove the cancer. Medical centers that have extensive experience with prostate surgery also tend to produce better results.

External irradiation can eliminate the cancer for the remaining life of the patient while avoiding some of the immediate postoperative side effects. It has its own risks, including diarrhea from radiation-induced inflammation of the rectum in the short term and chronic radiation injury to the rectum and gradual decline of sexual function over the long term. Newer conformal radiation therapy employs carefully shaped beams to maximize the destruction of cancer cells while limiting damage to surrounding tissue. The technique reduces the risk of bowel damage to about one in 100 and that of impotence to about one in three. The National Cancer Institute's consensus conference on prostate cancer, held in 1987, concluded that the survival rates for surgery and for radiation were indistinguishable at both five and 10 years after treatment.

Watchful waiting, the most conservative option, avoids treatment-related risks, but it subjects a man to constant anxiety about progression of his cancer and the possibility of a protracted, painful death. Such conservative treatment does not imply postponing therapy but rather a deliberate decision to forgo attempts to cure the cancer in the belief that a patient may well die of old age or some other cause before the malignancy leads to debility or death. Such patients should expect to need palliative treatment, including hormones or radiotherapy, if the cancer progresses. Some studies have suggested that no treatment results in survival rates equal to those of surgery or of radiation, but those studies all suffer from flaws that make them inconclusive [see "The Dilemmas of Prostate

Cancer," by Marc B. Garnick; SCIENTIFIC AMERICAN, April 1994].

Cancerous prostate tissue can also be treated by cryotherapy (insertion of a probe cooled with liquid nitrogen) or interstitial seed implantation, which employs tiny radioactive pellets whose intense radiation does not penetrate far enough to reach other tissue. Not enough is known thus far about the side effects or success rates of either method to permit comparison with established therapies.

PSA testing has revolutionized our understanding of prostate cancer and led to a dramatic increase in its detection. As a result, prostate cancers are being detected far earlier than before, at a time when most cancers can be treated with a high probability of cure. Nevertheless, such screening, and the treatment of tumors once detected, remains among the most controversial subjects in medicine.

Appropriate studies to determine the value of PSA testing in reducing the overall rate of death from prostate cancer—or in extending life in general (given that so many prostate patients die of other causes)—have simply not been done. Some large, long-term randomized trials and studies of easily tracked populations are now under way, including the NCI's Prostate, Lung, Colon and Ovarian Cancer Screening Trial. Even so, results will not be available for at least 10 years. Until then, men must decide for themselves whether the potential life-extending benefits of PSA screening and treatment outweigh the risks.

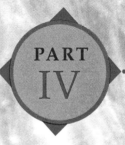

# IMPROVING
# CONVENTIONAL
# THERAPY

The mainstays of cancer treatment—
surgery, radiation and chemotherapy—
are being refined and combined in ways
that can help patients enjoy longer, more
fulfilling lives.

# Advancing Current Treatments for Cancer

*Surgery, radiation and chemotherapy can now cure many cases of cancer.*
*Future methods will be even more effective.*

• • •

Samuel Hellman and Everett E. Vokes

People often express hope for a cure for cancer—as though cancer sufferers never recover. In fact, most patients with skin cancer and about half the people treated for internal cancers are completely freed of their disease. But the longing for a cure that echoes throughout society reflects a legitimate dissatisfaction with current treatments. The therapies now available for internal tumors often give rise to side effects so harmful that they compromise the benefits of treatment. Existing therapies for such internal cancers can also fail in many cases, a sad reality that forces physicians to quote survival statistics to their patients instead of providing solid assurances of a recovery.

The situation should be much better. Cures for cancer should be more like the antibiotics physicians administer for infectious diseases. Anticancer treatments should be safe, effective and discriminating. Their actions should be limited to cancer cells and should result in few, if any, side effects. Most important, treatment should consistently return the patient to his or her former state of health. The ground has been broken for constructing such ideal remedies, but the completion of these ambitious projects will require medical researchers to deepen their understanding of the mechanisms that underlie various forms of cancer.

## Current Treatments for Cancer

Cancer is not a single disease. Rather it encompasses a large group of highly varied disorders that share certain key characteristics. Three of the features common to the many different cancers give rise to their most deleterious effects. The first and most fundamental quality of cancerous tissue is its continued enlargement (often the cause of the patient's symptoms) through the ability of cancer cells to proliferate indefinitely. Associated with this uncontrolled cell growth and division is the invasion of the tumor into surrounding normal tissue. Lastly, there is the most feared aspect of cancer: its tendency to spread throughout the body when cancer cells break away from the primary tumor, voyage through the circulatory system and establish colonies at distant sites—the process of metastasis. Most current cancer treatments aim to combat uncontrolled growth, tissue invasion and metastasis.

The earliest therapy established for cancer—and still the most widely used approach—is surgery.

# Treating Cancer with Radiation

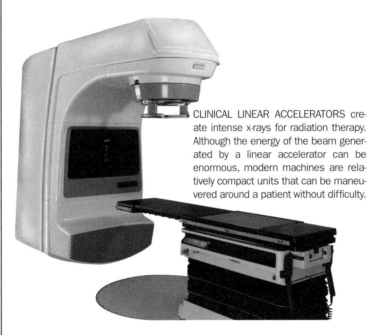

CLINICAL LINEAR ACCELERATORS create intense x-rays for radiation therapy. Although the energy of the beam generated by a linear accelerator can be enormous, modern machines are relatively compact units that can be maneuvered around a patient without difficulty.

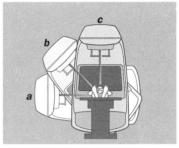

ROTATION of the linear accelerator around the patient allows the beam to irradiate the tumor from different directions. Variation of the path traversed by the x-ray beam concentrates the radiation in the tumor and so minimizes damage to surrounding healthy tissue.

CONFORMAL RADIOTHERAPY requires that the shape and direction of the x-ray beam change continually. For example, in applying radiation to treat prostate cancer, the shape of the beam varies to match the outline of the prostate (*yellow*), whether the beam is directed from the side (*a*), from an oblique angle (*b*) or from the front (*c*). Adjacent organs, such as the colon (*pink*) and bladder (*orange*), are thus spared unnecessary irradiation. In some facilities, a computerized mechanism sculpts the beam (*insets below*) by adjusting the position of a set of metal fingers in the aperture of the linear accelerator. The result is to deposit most of the therapeutic radiation (*red area, right*) where the target appears on a computed tomographic scan (*black outline, right*).

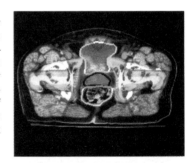

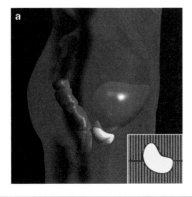

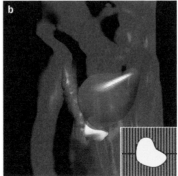

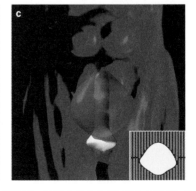

Surgical excision of a tumor is both quick and effective, and it accounts for the largest number of cures. Surgery is also the one method of therapy that offers the opportunity to confirm that a tumor has been fully excised, because a pathologist can examine the specimen removed (which should contain a layer of unaltered cells fully surrounding the cancerous ones).

Unfortunately, this form of treatment has several critical shortcomings. Removal of the tumor mass visible to the surgeon does not in itself guarantee elimination of the microscopic extensions that so often characterize cancer. To fully encompass this invasive edge around a tumor, a surgeon may be forced to cut out a large amount of healthy tissue and in doing so may severely damage the patient's functioning or appearance. Sometimes cancer grips vital structures that cannot be surgically removed. Even when surgery is possible, major operations (and the general anesthesia required for them) invariably traumatize patients. Perhaps the most crucial limitation of surgery is that it cannot treat cancer that has metastasized widely throughout the body.

Radiation therapy is preferable to surgery in many instances (see the box "Treating Cancer with radiation"). With this method, powerful x-rays or gamma rays (delivered by using an externally applied beam or, in some instances, by implanting tiny radioactive sources) irradiate the region of the patient's cancerous tumor. Radiation treatments act either by inflicting genetic damage sufficient to kill cells directly or by inducing cellular suicide, a process called apoptosis, which is deeply ingrained in mammalian cells. (Apoptosis is especially important during the embryonic development of mammals, when structures, such as gills, arise but then are lost as the cells constituting them undergo programmed cell death.)

Because healthy tissues can recover from radiation exposure more readily than cancerous cells, radiation therapy can preserve the anatomical structures that surround a cancerous growth, thus curing the cancer without sacrificing the patient's ability to function. Cancer of the uterine cervix and the early stages of both prostate cancer and Hodgkin's disease are well treated with radiation therapy. This technique is also especially important for treating cancer of the larynx (voice box), which can be cured without impairing the patient's ability to speak.

In addition to preserving normal tissue, radiation therapy has other advantages over surgical removal of a tumor. Radiation can, for instance, destroy microscopic extensions of cancerous tissue around a tumor that a scalpel might miss. Radiation is a safer option for older, frailer patients who might have difficulty recovering from surgery. Patients treated with radiation routinely receive five to eight weeks of daily treatments without requiring hospitalization.

Despite these many attractive attributes, radiation therapy at times proves inadequate, because it—like surgery—sometimes fails to eradicate all the cancer cells of a tumor. And like surgery, radiation cannot treat widespread metastases that will eventually form full-fledged tumors at numerous sites. (Whole-body radiation exposure sufficient to kill widely dispersed cancer cells would destroy some delicate tissues that are vital.) In such cases, a patient must make use of chemotherapy, the systemic administration of anticancer drugs that travel throughout the body via the blood circulatory system. Many different compounds are currently in use as anticancer agents, and additional ones are constantly being screened and tested (see the box "Families of Chemotherapeutic Drugs"). Chemotherapeutic drugs typically operate on human cells much as do some antibiotics on bacteria: they prevent cells from multiplying by interfering with their ability to replicate DNA. In at least some cases, anticancer drugs (like radiation treatment) appear to induce apoptosis in cancerous cells.

The first chemotherapeutic drugs, developed during the 1940s, often proved inadequate when administered individually or even in sequence. But during the 1960s, physicians discovered that chemotherapy could cure some cancers when several drugs were given at the same time. Many malignancies— leukemias, lymphomas and testicular cancer—are now successfully treated by such combination chemotherapy. Such cures are particularly meaningful because these cancers frequently strike young people, who stand to gain many more years of life than typical cancer patients do. Unfortunately, the majority of the most common cancers (breast, lung, colorectal and prostate cancer) are not yet curable with chemotherapy alone. For these conditions, chemotherapy can serve only as one component in an overall program of care that may also involve surgery and radiation.

The available chemotherapeutic drugs often fail patients because they kill many healthy cells and thus bring on serious side effects that limit the doses physicians can administer. Damage to the rapidly growing cells of the bone marrow, for instance, causes anemia, an inability to fight infection and a propensity for internal bleeding, because the

# Families of Chemotherapeutic Drugs

## ANTIMETABOLITES

Some anticancer compounds act as false substances in the biochemical reactions of a living cell. A prime example of such a drug is methotrexate, which is a chemical analogue for the nutrient folic acid. Methotrexate functions, in part, by binding to an enzyme (*orange*) normally involved in the conversion of folic acid into two of the building blocks of DNA, adenine and guanine. This drug thus prevents cells from dividing by incapacitating their ability to construct new DNA.

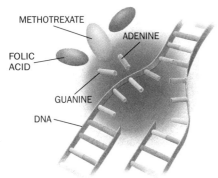

Examples: methotrexate, fluorouracil, gemcitabine

## TOPOISOMERASE INHIBITORS

Replication of a cell's genetic material requires a means to pull the DNA double helix apart into two strands. This separation is typically accomplished with the aid of a special "topoisomerase" enzyme (*orange*) that temporarily cleaves one strand, passes the other strand through the break and then reattaches the cut ends together. Drugs that inhibit the ability of topoisomerase enzymes to reattach the broken ends cause pervasive DNA strand breaks in cells that are dividing, a process that causes these cells to die.

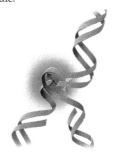

Examples: doxorubicin, CPT-11

## ALKYLATING AGENTS

Certain compounds (*orange*) form chemical bonds with particular DNA building blocks and so produce defects in the normal double helical structure of the DNA molecule. This disruption may take the form of breaks and inappropriate links between (or within) strands. If not mended by the various DNA repair mechanisms available to the cell, the damage caused by these chemicals will trigger cellular suicide.

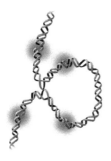

Examples: cyclophosphamide, chlorambucil

## PLANT ALKALOIDS

Certain substances derived from plants can prevent cell division by binding to the protein tubulin. Tubulin, as its name implies, forms microtubular fibers (*pink*) that help to orchestrate cell division. These fibers pull duplicated DNA chromosomes to either side of the parental cell, ensuring that each daughter cell receives a full set of genetic blueprints. Drugs that interfere with the assembly or disassembly of these tubulin fibers can prevent cells from dividing successfully.

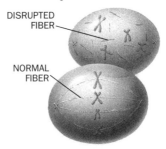

Examples: vinblastine, vinorelbine, paclitaxel, docetaxel

patient cannot produce an adequate number of red blood cells, white blood cells and platelets (the cells responsible for clotting). Other side effects of chemotherapy include diarrhea, nausea, vomiting and hair loss. Less commonly, these drugs may damage the nervous system.

Although strategies for ameliorating many of these unwanted side effects are quickly evolving, chemotherapy as currently offered retains another fundamental weakness. Like bacteria resistant to antibiotics, some tumors are able to survive the anticancer drugs used to treat them. Certain tumors prove to be drug resistant from the outset, whereas others develop resistance with repeated treatment. The problem of drug resistance in chemotherapy is particularly serious because tumors can develop a resistance to multiple drugs after only one drug has been administered to the patient. Another kind of drug therapy, available for some cancers, sidesteps many of the difficulties associated with chemotherapy. The alternative scheme works by manipulating the body's endocrine system. The breast and prostate are glands regulated by sex hormones, and malignancies that arise from those tissues may also respond to these hormones. This sensitivity can be exploited: physicians can administer antiestrogens to women with breast cancer, and they can give drugs that provide a so-called androgen blockade for men with prostate cancer. Such hormone therapy has relatively mild side effects, because its actions are limited largely to tissues with receptors for specific hormones. Hormone therapy is, however, valuable only to patients with tumors of these particular tissues. And even with people so afflicted, this approach sometimes proves ineffective, because tumors of the breast and prostate may contain some hormone-independent cells that can still proliferate dangerously.

## Combining Different Treatments

Physicians can categorize most solid tumors at the time of initial diagnosis according to extent of progression. In general, small tumors that have not spread to lymph nodes or other distant sites are denoted as being in stage one. Stage-two and stage-three tumors are more advanced, being larger and involving more lymph nodes. Stage-four tumors have progressed to the point of establishing readily detectable metastases elsewhere in the body.

Physicians use surgery or radiotherapy to destroy early-stage tumors at their primary sites and,

if necessary, in nearby lymph nodes. For patients with stage-four tumors, the prognosis is usually grim, and caregivers typically devise therapies aimed only at reducing the person's immediate symptoms and at extending survival. (Chemotherapy usually serves these aims in such advanced cases.) Therapy for intermediate stages of cancer is difficult to categorize simply, and its methods of treatment are changing the most swiftly. Patients with intermediate-stage tumors can often be cured, having all traces of their cancer completely eliminated. Yet many patients will experience only a temporary remission before recurrence of cancer because microscopic tumor deposits (rogue cells that were present but undiscovered at the time of initial diagnosis) will ultimately grow out of control.

For people with intermediate-stage cancers, physicians increasingly employ various mixtures of distinct treatments in so-called combined modality therapy. Combined modality therapy can demand the efforts of a wide assortment of specialists—oncologists, surgeons, pathologists and radiologists—and the coordination of this care often poses a logistical challenge.

The most common combination of cancer treatments is surgery or radiotherapy followed up with chemotherapy. Perhaps the best example of this approach is found in the current treatment of breast cancer. Surgical removal of the tumor and a small amount of surrounding tissue (a procedure called lumpectomy), when combined with radiation and drug therapy, has improved the cure rate of breast cancer and has made removal of the breast unnecessary in most cases. A similar strategy has also been shown to increase the rate of cure for colorectal cancer and for some cancers of bone and soft tissue.

A newer form of combined modality therapy—induction chemotherapy—applies chemotherapy first and surgery or radiotherapy afterward. This procedure allows an oncologist to gauge the effectiveness of the chemotherapeutic drugs by observing how fast the primary tumor shrinks.

Induction chemotherapy permits treatment of tumor cells disseminated throughout the body—systemic micrometastases—as early as possible. In some cases, it may reduce or even eliminate the need for organ-removing surgery. For example, patients with advanced cancers of the head and neck have traditionally been treated with surgery and radiotherapy, yet they often succumbed to the disease. Those patients who survived radical surgical procedures were sometimes left unable to speak. Induction chemotherapy followed by radiotherapy can achieve similar survival rates without producing this devastating impairment. Physicians have similarly used induction chemotherapy successfully to treat cancer of the lung and bladder; in the latter case, this therapy often renders removal of the bladder unnecessary. Induction hormone therapy, with later radiation or surgery, can also be quite effective in treating prostate cancer.

Chemotherapy or hormonal therapy can also be administered at the same time as surgery or radiotherapy. This approach, known as concomitant chemoradiotherapy, is particularly valuable for treating tumors that are likely to respond poorly to surgery or radiotherapy alone (that is, tumors that would most probably survive these treatments or have already metastasized). The treatment of cancer of the esophagus, for example, has been shown to be more successful with concomitant chemoradiotherapy than with radiotherapy alone. The addition of chemotherapy in these cases reduces the chance that the cancer will later return to that region of the body or develop in some other organ.

## Future Prospects

New surgical techniques involving tiny incisions and special instruments that let surgeons see and operate deep within a patient's body are becoming more frequently applied in cancer therapy (see Figure 8.1). These methods should help spare some cancer patients the trauma of traditional surgery. But the largest strides in cancer treatment will undoubtedly derive from advances in radiation therapy and chemotherapy that increase the effectiveness of these methods in killing cancer cells without causing permanent damage to healthy tissues.

Some gains may take many years to become routinely available to cancer patients, but others appear to be on the threshold of widespread application.

Radiation therapy, for instance, is improving rapidly as medical practitioners grow increasingly able to tailor each treatment to the circumstances of the patient's cancer. In particular, technological innovations now allow therapists to manipulate external beams of radiation so as to target the tumor precisely, avoiding harm to surrounding tissues (see the box "Treating Cancer with Radiation"). Such techniques go under the banner of conformal radiotherapy, because the beam of radiation conforms closely to the shape of the tumor.

Conformal radiotherapy requires an array of advanced technology. First, the three-dimensional configuration of the tumor must be ascertained by computed tomographic x-ray scans or magnetic resonance imaging. This information, recorded digitally, becomes the basis for a detailed treatment plan that specifies the direction and shape of the beam (as well as the intensity and duration of the irradiation). That plan maximizes the dose of radiation absorbed by the tumor while minimizing the exposure of the surrounding tissue. The prescribed radiation treatment is then delivered under computer control using a linear accelerator, a relatively compact instrument that can generate high-intensity x-rays yet still be maneuvered readily around the patient.

Conformal radiotherapy lets a collaborating team of physicians, radiation physicists and therapists safely increase the dose—and with it the likelihood of cure—administered to prostate tumors without raising (and, in fact, sometimes reducing) the injury done to disease-free tissue. Groups of medical researchers are also applying this technique

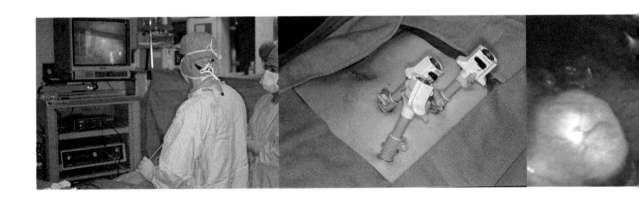

experimentally to many other localized tumors and even to multiple metastases in those special circumstances when only a few metastases occur. Another emerging technique in conformal radiotherapy treats brain tumors by using a special frame affixed directly to the patient's cranium. By aiming the x-ray source with respect to the rigid frame, technicians can position the beam extremely precisely during each treatment.

Although x-rays and gamma rays are the mainstays of radiation therapy, protons and neutrons also work well. Protons target tumor-bearing sites better than x-rays do, and neutrons seem to have more potency against some cancers. It remains to be seen how effective these particles will ultimately prove, but recent studies suggest real promise for treating certain types of cancer. Protons can, for example, treat small tumors of the spine that lie near vital structures, and neutrons work effectively on salivary gland tumors.

Improvements in chemotherapy will come with the advent of new drugs. Exciting anticancer compounds recently introduced for clinical use include the yew tree–derived taxanes, which are effective for treating advanced ovarian and breast cancers [see "Taxoids: New Weapons against Cancer," by K. C. Nicolaou, Rodney K. Guy and Pierre Potier; SCIENTIFIC AMERICAN, June 1996]. The so-called camptothecan derivatives are showing promise in patients with colorectal and lung cancer. Both types of drugs have mechanisms of action that distinguish them from older chemotherapeutic agents. Procedural changes in the administration of chemotherapeutic drugs may also bring higher rates of cure. For example, prolonged intravenous infusion using implanted pumps can expose a tumor to a drug over a longer period of growth and vulnerability, yielding better results (see Figure 8.2).

Some current efforts at improving chemotherapy are focused on combating drug resistance. Still other drug therapies on the horizon might operate by preventing tumors from establishing an adequate blood supply or by enlisting the body's immune system to fight tumors (see Part V, "Therapies of the Future"). New "differentiating" agents are also in early clinical trials. Rather than killing tumor cells, these drugs cause cancer cells to undergo so-called terminal differentiation—that is, the cells give up their ability to divide and commit themselves to carrying out a single function, not unlike most cells of the body. Differentiating agents offer a form of chemotherapy that is much less toxic than are current cell-killing drugs.

Physicians have recently made great headway in reducing toxic side effects and improving supportive care for people undergoing chemotherapy. For instance, new and more powerful drugs to prevent vomiting have helped these patients. Because chemotherapy typically damages the rapidly dividing cells lining the alimentary system, diarrhea and oral sensitivity are common side effects. New drugs that stimulate the growth and repair of these lining cells may soon be available to treat the cause of this toxicity—not just the symptoms.

Researchers have recently experimented with various growth factors that can stimulate the blood precursor cells in the bone marrow to recover quickly after chemotherapy. Drugs that increase white blood cell production, for instance, help to protect patients from severe complicating infections. One drug in development has been shown to stimulate the bone marrow to produce platelets that aid in blood clotting. Moreover, a strategy for

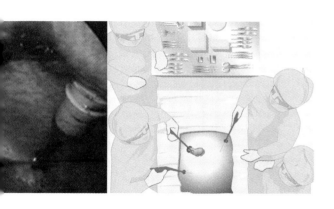

Figure 8.1 COLON SURGERY has traditionally required a large incision to open the patient's abdomen fully, but laparoscopically assisted operations now allow colon cancer to be treated with far less trauma to the patient. Physicians at the Mayo Clinic and several other institutions are currently conducting clinical trials of this procedure (*far left*), whereby surgical instruments penetrate small holes in the abdominal wall (*left of center*). While monitoring video images of the inside of the patient's inflated abdomen, surgeons detach a section of bowel from the side of the abdominal wall (*right of center*). They can then bring part of the bowel outside the body through a small incision and remove the cancerous segment (*far right*).

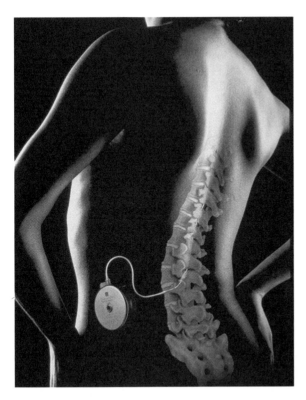

**Figure 8.2 IMPLANTABLE PUMPS, placed under the skin in a patient's abdomen or chest, allow chemotherapeutic drugs and narcotics to be infused continuously, thereby helping to relieve some chronic, intractable cancer pain.**

administering high-dose treatments while protecting blood precursor cells is becoming widely used for cancers that physicians cannot cure with conventional levels of chemotherapy (see the following "Current Controversy: When Are Bone Marrow Transplants Considered?").

One must not underestimate the ability of early detection of cancer to improve cure rates by allowing a tumor to be treated when it is smaller, less aggressive and less likely to have metastasized. Physicians have made good progress in using medical imaging for detecting cancer. The modern understanding of the genetic basis of cancer is providing the means to test for inborn susceptibility to certain cancers, to give early warnings of its occurrence in some cases and to gauge its severity after it arises.

## More Definitive Therapies

Much of this book is devoted to the expanding body of knowledge about the molecular and genetic basis of cancer. This newly gained understanding should eventually spawn more effective therapies for treating cancer and, ultimately, strategies for cancer prevention. In the nearer term, physicians should be able to use molecular and genetic markers to determine the malignancy potential of tumors and their likelihood of responding to different treatments.

Gene therapy opens a new arena for cancer treatment. With our colleagues at the University of Chicago we are pursuing the possibility of combining radiation and gene therapy, so as to use the radiation beam to trigger the production of proteins toxic to cancer cells at specific sites in the body. We have carried out this rather remarkable feat in experimental animals by introducing into cancerous tissue a "radiation-inducible" gene, one that is specially engineered to switch on (that is, to allow manufacture of the protein that it encodes) only after it has been exposed to radiation. This technique—called regional gene therapy—should greatly increase the effectiveness and specificity of radiation in treating cancer. It will enter clinical trials shortly.

## A War Half Won

War often serves as a metaphor for cancer research. Although the analogy can at times be misleading, it can also illuminate the current position of medical researchers. During World War II, there was a period before D-Day when substantial advances had been made by the Allies, but a true offensive had not begun. Looking at the map, one might have thought the gains in Africa or Italy were minimal. But extraordinary improvements in weapons, personnel and the means to deliver them together to western Europe had been largely worked out.

Although some modest advances in the treatment of cancer have been made, these limited successes do not reveal the tremendous developments in the tools medical researchers and practitioners have at their fingertips. It is difficult at this moment to predict how useful any specific discovery will be, but the cumulative benefits to cancer therapy can be assured. Yet it is important to keep expectations realistic. A simple, universal treatment that is effective for all cancers, while possible, is extremely unlikely to emerge anytime in the near future. But a large set of more specific and less toxic treatments is probably nearer at hand than most people might think.

# Current Controversy: When Are Bone Marrow Transplants Considered?

...

Karen Antman

Every year doctors in the United States tell thousands of patients that a bone marrow transplant, and not conventional therapy, may eradicate their disease. The side effects of such a transplant-which for some cancers is still experimental-can be substantial, even lethal. Nevertheless, a relatively young and otherwise healthy person faced with a deadly disease will often opt for this chance to be cured.

At one time, the term "bone marrow transplant" did indeed refer to the marrow found within cavities of the bone; today, however, the term often denotes a "stem cell transplant." Marrow is rich in hematopoietic, or blood-forming, stem cells, primitive cells that multiply and metamorphose into the different components of blood: red cells, which carry oxygen; white cells, which fight infection; and platelets, which help blood to clot. Although some stem cells also circulate in the blood, they reside primarily in the marrow, where they generate a soup of developing blood cells [see "The Stem Cell," by David W. Golde; SCIENTIFIC AMERICAN, December 1991].

Bone marrow can, however, become diseased by aplastic anemia, a condition in which marrow, having degenerated into scar tissue, produces too few blood cells; by leukemia, a disease characterized literally by "too many in blood" (emia) "white" (leuk) cells; or by several other disorders. Chemotherapy and radiation, widely used for treating diverse cancers, can also harm marrow. Because blood cells made in the marrow are responsible for fighting bacteria, viruses and other invaders and for causing blood to clot, damaged marrow results in a high risk of death from infection or bleeding, or both.

When the marrow itself is diseased, a transplant is intended to replace it with healthy blood-forming tissue supplied by a donor. In other cases, a bone marrow transplant is done to compensate for the toxic effects of unusually intense chemotherapy. These high levels of drugs kill not only cancer cells but also other fast-growing cells such as those generating blood or hair or lining the mouth, stomach or intestines. The resulting side effects, such as hair loss, nausea or diarrhea, can be unpleasant or

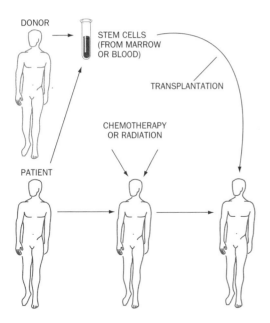

DONOR

STEM CELLS
(FROM MARROW
OR BLOOD)

TRANSPLANTATION

CHEMOTHERAPY
OR RADIATION

PATIENT

**TRANSPLANT PROCEDURE begins with the patient or donor providing stem cells. These blood-forming cells are stored while the patient's malignant cells are killed. The stem cells are then returned to the patient to speed the recovery of bone marrow.**

worse; most seriously, however, a patient without enough blood cells would die of infection or bleeding within a few weeks. Transplant of stem cells after chemotherapy helps to speed recovery of the blood supply.

To begin a transplant, doctors first collect stem cells from a donor or from the patient (see the Figure "Transplant Procedure"). The stem cells may come from the marrow, or they may be extracted directly from the blood. The patient is then given high levels of radiation or drugs to destroy any cancerous cells. Afterward, the stem cells are injected into the bloodstream; they home to the bony cavities and settle there, regenerating the marrow. Reseeded with stem cells collected from the blood, marrow generally recovers in two weeks, but recovery takes five weeks if the stem cells come from the marrow itself. (Researchers suspect that some of the stem cells in the blood are more mature and so take less time to complete their development.) Consequently, fewer patients transplanted with stem cells from blood die in the vulnerable period following the treatment, when the blood cells are still too sparse to ward off infec-

tions. Unfortunately, because circulating blood sometimes cannot supply enough stem cells for a full transplant, marrow may have to be used.

For a patient whose marrow is diseased, a brother, sister or unrelated person with a matching tissue type may be able to donate stem cells, enabling what is called an allogeneic transplant. But even if the major indicators of tissue type—as measured by a procedure called human leukocyte antigen (HLA) typing—signal a perfect match, there may still be minor mismatches. In that case, the immune cells generated by the donated stem cells might recognize the host tissue as foreign and attack it, primarily damaging the skin, bowel and liver. The risk of this complication, called graft versus host disease (GVHD), increases if the marrow comes from an unrelated donor. The risk is also considerably higher for older patients.

To test for the likelihood of GVHD, a doctor will typically mix a few donor cells with tissue from the recipient; only donors whose cells have no reaction are accepted. Even so, serious GVHD occurs about half the time, leading to death in about 20 to 30 percent of recipients of allogeneic tissue—or in a higher percentage of patients if the tissues match imperfectly. Oddly enough, however, mild or moderate GVHD can be beneficial to leukemia patients. The new immune cells also attack the cancerous leukemia cells, resulting in a graft versus leukemia (GVL) effect and thereby reducing the risk of a relapse.

In the unlikely event that a patient has an identical twin, he or she can donate stem cells that are perfectly matched, in a procedure called a syngeneic transplant. These cells are safe in that they cannot cause GVHD. (But syngeneic transplants also cannot give rise to GVL, and thus recipients run a high risk of relapse.) Hematopoietic stem cells can also be obtained from the placenta and umbilical cord discarded after a baby is born: such "cord blood transplants" appear to pose a lower risk of GVHD. But whereas the number of stem cells obtained from a placenta are enough to perform transplantation on a child, they may be too few for an adult.

The most common form of marrow transplant done today is an autologous transplant, in which the stem cells come from the patient, having been withdrawn before chemotherapy. Because marrow obtained from the patient is perfectly matched, there is no risk of GVHD. Unfortunately, marrow from a cancer patient may be contaminated by tumor cells, which at least in theory may cause a relapse (in practice one cannot tell if a cancer recurred because marrow was contaminated or because some cancerous cells in the body survived chemotherapy). But overall, autologous transplant patients have the lowest risk of death from complications. For breast cancer, the mortality for the procedure is generally between 1 and 7 percent; for lymphomas, it is about 10 percent.

Marrow transplants are standard for a few cancers (see the figure "Marrow Transplants") but available in research studies for many. To treat some cancers, doctors usually choose to perform the procedure if the patient can tolerate it. For example, the only curative treatment for chronic myeloid leukemia, in which the white blood cells that fight bacteria are diseased, is an allogeneic bone marrow transplant. An allogeneic transplant is often preferred for patients with severe aplastic anemia or myelodysplasia (a condition marked by abnormal marrow cells, often degenerating to aplastic anemia or leukemia).

High-dose chemotherapy or radiation, combined with autologous transplants, is beneficial for treating myeloma, recurring Hodgkin's disease or aggressive non-Hodgkin's lymphoma (malignancies of the lymph system). Advanced or recurring testicular cancer and neuroblastoma—a childhood cancer that after a certain point cannot be cured by conventional chemotherapy—also respond to such a combination of intensive therapy and a stem cell transplant.

In some other cancers, initial results with the therapy-and-transplant regimen have been promising but remain controversial. In North America, most marrow transplants are prescribed for breast cancer. For women whose cancer has metastasized, conventional chemotherapy can keep the disease in check for several years, occasionally a decade or more; however, virtually all such patients eventually succumb to it. Data from the Autologous Blood and Marrow Transplant Registry of North America show that five years after a marrow transplant, between 15 and 20 percent of the women were still in remission. Physicians are concerned that these results might have been skewed by selection of relatively healthy women for the transplants. But one small randomized clinical trial conducted in South Africa also reported in 1995 an improved, three-year survival rate for breast cancer patients who

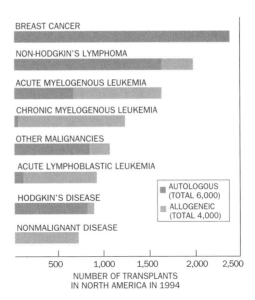

MARROW TRANSPLANTS are most often used for treating breast cancer, even though the efficacy of this application is controversial. The transplants are, on the other hand, known to be beneficial for treating several cancers involving blood or lymph cells.

underwent marrow transplants as compared with those who received conventional chemotherapy.

Still, the paucity of randomized data on the effectiveness of bone marrow transplants for breast cancer makes this treatment one of the most contentious issues in modern medicine. More than 10 large-scale randomized trials are currently under way, some of which examine transplants for treating locally advanced breast cancers as well as metastasized malignancies. But American researchers are having trouble recruiting enough patients for these trials. Some women do not want to risk being in the control group—and thus not receiving what they consider to be the best treatment. At the same time, some women do not wish to receive a transplant if it is not known to be a better option. The uncertainties of the procedure, however, can be resolved only if the clinical trials can be completed.

For some other cancers, patients with little chance of survival through conventional treatments can obtain high-dose chemotherapy with a marrow transplant in research studies. These diseases include ovarian cancer and brain tumors.

Recent research has raised hopes of alleviating one risk from bone marrow transplants. An article in the August 3, 1995, *New England Journal of Medicine* describes how scientists are starting with small amounts of marrow cells and attempting to grow them in the laboratory so that the patient can be given both stem cells and mature cells. This combination would eliminate the period during which he or she is at risk from infections. At present, however, given that the side effects remain daunting, a patient should choose a bone marrow transplant only when the disease is life-threatening and when the potential benefits exceed the expected risk. Even so, to some patients with little to hope for, bone marrow transplants do offer a new lease on life.

# Fact Sheet: Twelve Major Cancers

. . .

The pages that follow provide facts and figures about the 12 cancers that affect the most Americans (excluding basal cell and squamous cell skin cancers, which are very common but rarely fatal). Cancer is most successfully treated if detected early. For this reason, many physicians recommend that people over age 40 have annual health checkups, which can often catch disease before it produces any symptoms. (People between the ages of 20 and 40 should have checkups every three years.) People who do have any of the symptoms described are wise to consult a doctor. None of these symptoms prove that someone has cancer, however-a firm diagnosis can be made only by a trained oncologist. Readers wishing to learn about the latest research on particular cancers can find resources listed in the box "Finding More Information" at the end of Part VI, "Living With Cancer."

Certain characteristics are shared by virtually all cancers. The risk of the disease developing usually increases with advancing age. Curing a solid tumor—eliminating all traces of cancer from the body—generally becomes more difficult the larger the tumor has grown. Metastasis to distant body locations is more worrisome than local spreading or no spreading. (The extent of a cancer's spread is referred to as its stage.) In addition, examining detailed features of the tumor cells under a microscope is usually important in evaluating their aggressiveness.

Broad categories of cancer treatments include:

- **Surgery** to remove a tumor or diseased tissue. It is the primary mode of treatment for most solid tumors.

- **Chemotherapy,** the use of drugs to kill tumor cells. It, too, has a role in most cancer treatments. The several classes of chemotherapeutic drugs act by various means, most frequently by inhibiting the ability of tumor cells to replicate correctly. Many drugs are commonly used in combination because tumors may be unable to defend themselves against a variety of agents attacking in different ways. The compounds may be introduced into the body as a whole, or they may be concentrated at the tumor site.

- **Radiation** to kill tumor cells. Sometimes used as a primary form of treatment, it is more often an adjunct to other therapies. The radiation may be aimed at a tumor from outside the body, or it may be delivered by placing radioactive pellets or liquid at the cancerous site.

- **Biological therapies,** which are based on complex substances found in living organisms. They include immunotherapies, which attempt to turn the body's immune system against a cancer.

- **Hormone-blocking and hormone-supplementing therapies,** which affect the rate at which tumor cells grow, multiply or die.

- **Bone marrow transplantation,** which is not a therapy in itself but is sometimes used to strengthen the depleted blood-making system of a patient weakened by high, potentially curative doses of radiation or chemotherapies (see the preceding section "Current Controversy: When Are Bone Marrow Transplants Considered?"). Healthy cells for the transplants may come from other people (allogeneic donations) or from samples of blood or bone marrow collected previously from the patient (autologous donations).

Throughout, survival figures are expressed as relative rates. The numbers refer to the proportion of people with a disease who are expected to be alive at a later time, compared with a similar population that is free of cancer. If the five-year relative survival rate for a type of cancer is 50 percent, for instance, there will be half as many survivors in a group of patients as in a comparable cancer-free group. Relative survival thus reflects mortality from the cancer alone, correcting for deaths from other illnesses or accidents. Sadly, survival five years after diagnosis does not equate with a cure. Some intractable cancers continue to progress over extended periods, and others may recur after they seem to be eliminated.

*— The Editors* of
SCIENTIFIC AMERICAN

## PROSTATE CANCER

- **317,100 new cases to be diagnosed in the U.S. this year**
- **41,400 deaths expected**

*Prostate cancer is the second leading cause of cancer death in men.*

**Risk Factors:** Increasing age; possibly a high-fat diet. Prostate cancer may tend to run in families, but whether the cause is genetic or environmental is unclear. The incidence in black men is 37 percent higher than in white men, and the mortality rate is twice as high.

**Warning Signs:** Urine flow that is weak, interrupted or difficult to control; frequent need to urinate; painful urination; back or pelvic pain.

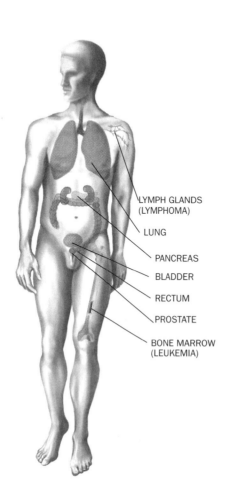

LYMPH GLANDS (LYMPHOMA)
LUNG
PANCREAS
BLADDER
RECTUM
PROSTATE
BONE MARROW (LEUKEMIA)

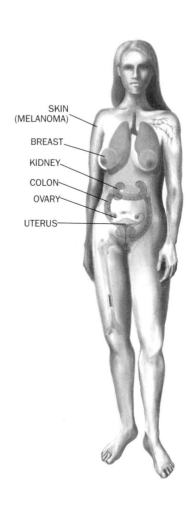

SKIN (MELANOMA)
BREAST
KIDNEY
COLON
OVARY
UTERUS

**Detection and Diagnosis:** Every man older than 50 years should have a digital rectal examination annually. A prostate-specific antigen (PSA) blood test can signal the presence of prostate abnormalities at an early stage. Transrectal ultrasound evaluation can confirm suspicious results from other tests. Examination of the amount of DNA in abnormal cells can indicate how aggressive a cancer may be.

*Under study:* Detailed genetic analysis of tumor cells may help predict their aggressiveness.

**Treatment Now:** Removal of the prostate gland is routine. Radiotherapy is also widely used as an alternative or supplement to prostatectomy. Against metastatic disease, drugs can block cancer cells from receiving the male hormones they need to grow.

*Under study:* Radiation therapy with beams that are controlled so as to maximize radiation dose to the tumor with the smallest amount of collateral exposure. Radiation therapy in combination with hormones. Finasteride, a drug used to relieve symptoms caused by benign enlargement of the prostate, may prevent cancer.

**Five-Year Survival Rates:**

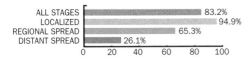

**Controversies:** The merits of PSA testing for detecting asymptomatic disease and the best approach for handling localized tumors are intensely debated (see the section "Current Controversy: Does Screening for Prostate Cancer Make Sense?," following Chapter 7).

## BREAST CANCER

- **185,700 new cases to be diagnosed in the U.S. this year (including 1,400 among men)**
- **44,560 deaths expected (including 260 men)**

*Breast cancer is the most common cancer among women.*

**Risk Factors:** Inherited mutations in the *BRCA1* or *BRCA2* genes; increasing age; early onset of menstruation; late menopause; never having had children or having a first child after age 30; personal or family history of breast cancer; possibly a

high-fat diet. Mortality rates are falling in white women, especially those younger than 65.

**Warning Signs:** A painless lump in the breast is typical, but there may occasionally be pain; any change in the shape, color or texture of the breast or nipple; discharge from or tenderness in the nipple.

**Detection and Diagnosis:** Self-examination and clinical breast exams; mammograms. Experts recommend annual mammograms and breast checkups for all women older than 50 but also for some younger women (see the section "Current Controversy: Should Women in Their 40s Have Mammograms?," following Chapter 7).

*Under study:* Biochemical and genetic markers and the density of blood vessels in a tumor may help indicate its aggressiveness.

**Treatment Now:** For localized tumors, mastectomy (removal of the whole breast) may be appropriate, but breast-conserving surgery (removal of the tumor and some surrounding tissue, sometimes called lumpectomy) followed by local radiation is often preferable. Although recurrences are more common with breast-conserving surgery, these can be treated by mastectomy, and the survival rates are equivalent to those when mastectomy is used initially. Either procedure may be followed by additional chemotherapy or hormone-blocking therapy. If tumor cells have high levels of receptors for the hormones estrogen and progesterone, it is a good sign because hormone-blocking therapy may stop their growth.

*Under study:* High-dose chemotherapy followed by reconstitution of damaged bone marrow; chemotherapy before surgery; immunotherapy, including immunotoxins (molecules that combine a toxic agent with an antibody that binds to tumor cells); new chemotherapies and drug combinations. Tamoxifen, a drug that suppresses the effects of estrogen, may help prevent breast cancer in some women at high risk.

**Five-Year Survival Rates:**

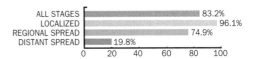

**Controversies:** Tests for detecting inherited mutations in the *BRCA1* and *BRCA2* genes are becoming available, but doctors have not reached a consensus on their use. Also debated are the value of chemotherapy for elderly patients and the value of routine mammography in women younger than 50. Some studies indicate that surgical treatment of breast cancer during the second half of a patient's menstrual cycle is more likely to produce a favorable outcome.

## LUNG CANCER

- **177,000 new cases to be diagnosed in the U.S. this year**
- **158,700 deaths expected**

*Incidence has been declining in men since the 1980s but is still rising in women.*

**Risk Factors:** Cigarette smoking (linked to 85 to 90 percent of all cases); exposure in the workplace to certain substances, including asbestos and some organic chemicals; radiation exposure; radon exposure (especially in smokers); environmental tobacco smoke.

**Warning Signs:** Persistent cough; sputum streaked with blood; wheezy breathing; chest or shoulder pain; swelling in face or neck; recurring pneumonia or bronchitis.

**Detection and Diagnosis:** Chest x-ray; analysis of cells in sputum; fiber-optic exam of the bronchial passages.

**Treatment Now:** Lung cancers are of two principal types, small cell or nonsmall cell disease. For small cell lung cancer, which spreads rapidly, chemotherapy alone or with radiation is now used instead of surgery. Radiation may be given to the chest or, in some cases, to the brain, to kill metastases. For localized nonsmall cell cancers, surgeons may remove the affected part of the lung, although recurrences are common. For more advanced cases, radiation, chemotherapy, laser therapy or some combination may be used instead.

*Under study:* Several new chemical agents (including taxol, taxotere, topotecan, irinotecan and vinorelbine) and biological agents (including interleukin-2 and interferon). Gene therapies are in clinical trials using "antisense" approaches to reestablish activity of the tumor suppressor protein p53 or to turn off oncogenes.

**Five-Year Survival Rates:**

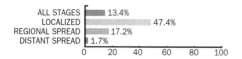

**Controversies:** The Food and Drug Administration is considering regulating cigarettes as drug-delivery devices, although any such move would face strong political opposition. Ventilation equipment can prevent radon, a naturally occurring radioactive gas, from accumulating in basements, but opinions vary about the value of this equipment in regions where radon levels are not exceptional.

## COLORECTAL CANCER

- **133,500 new cases to be diagnosed in the U.S. this year (94,500 for colon, 39,000 for rectum)**
- **54,900 deaths expected (46,400 for colon, 8,500 for rectum)**

**Risk Factors:** Family history of colorectal cancer; polyps or inflammatory bowel disease. Specific genetic mutations have been linked to familial adenomatous polyposis, which can develop into colon cancer, and hereditary nonpolyposis colorectal cancer. Living in an industrial or urban area also raises the risk. Other factors may include physical inactivity, exposure to certain chemicals and a high-fat or low-fiber diet.

**Warning Signs:** Blood in the stool; any change in bowel habits; general stomach discomfort; unaccountable weight loss.

**Detection and Diagnosis:** Annual digital rectal exam and stool blood test are recommended for people older than 40; sigmoidoscopy every three to five years after age 50. If possible problems are found, colonoscopy and a barium enema (to allow visualization of the intestines using x-rays) may be used. A patient's prognosis is poorer if the bowel is obstructed or perforated or if the pretreatment levels of certain marker substances (carcinoembryonic antigen and carbohydrate antigen 19-9) in the blood serum are high.

*Under study:* Various genetic tests looking at the *ras* oncogene, characteristic changes in colorectal cell DNA and mutations affecting DNA repair.

**Treatment Now:** Surgery to remove the tumor, sometimes combined with radiation or chemotherapy, or both. Occasionally, a colostomy may be necessary. If the disease has spread to the lymph nodes, chemotherapy with fluorouracil appears to be worthwhile. Chemotherapy combined with radiotherapy is used against intermediate and advanced rectal cancer. Surgical removal of metastases in the liver may prolong survival in some patients.

*Under study:* Combinations of chemotherapy and immunotherapy are under investigation for postoperative patients with cancerous lymph nodes, including the use of immunotoxins, which are molecules that combine a toxic agent with an antibody that binds to tumor cells. Biological therapy and surgery that spares a patient's sphincter are also being evaluated.

### Five-Year Survival Rates:

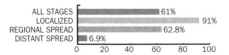

| | |
|---|---|
| ALL STAGES | 61% |
| LOCALIZED | 91% |
| REGIONAL SPREAD | 62.8% |
| DISTANT SPREAD | 6.9% |

0  20  40  60  80  100

**Controversies:** The benefit of chemotherapy without evidence of lymph node involvement is uncertain. The value of radiation in advanced cases is under study. To treat liver metastases, implantable drug pumps and infusion ports are sometimes used, but their worth is unproved.

## BLADDER CANCER

- **52,900 new cases to be diagnosed in the U.S. this year**
- **11,700 deaths expected**

**Risk Factors:** Whites get bladder cancer twice as often as blacks do, and men two to three times as often as women do. This cancer develops two to three times more often in cigarette smokers than in nonsmokers. Workers in the rubber, chemical and leather industries are at higher risk, as are hairdressers, machinists, metal workers, printers, painters, textile workers and truck drivers.

**Warning Signs:** Blood in urine; pain during urination; urgent or frequent need to urinate.

**Detection and Diagnosis:** A tumor can sometimes be felt during a rectal or vaginal examination. Cancer cells are sometimes seen in urine samples under a microscope. Cytoscopy (examination of the bladder with an instrument inserted in the urethra) can reveal abnormal areas. Biopsy is needed to confirm diagnosis.

*Under study:* Mutations in the *p53* gene that might signal tumor aggressiveness; changes in certain proteins found in cell nuclei.

**Treatment Now:** Early-stage cancer confined to the bladder wall can often be removed with a

cytoscope. If several tumors are present, doctors may remove them and then infuse the bladder with a solution containing bacteria able to stimulate the immune system. Chemotherapeutic drugs may also be put directly into the bladder to lower the risk of recurrence.

If the cancer cannot be easily removed, radiation (from an external source or from a radioisotope placed in the bladder) may be needed. If the cancer has spread through the bladder wall, the bladder may be removed. Chemotherapy may be needed after metastasis.

*Under study:* Bladder-sparing surgery with chemotherapy; interferon or interleukin-2 therapy for early-stage disease; photodynamic therapy (using laser light and a photosensitizer to kill tumor cells); the analysis of DNA alterations and proteins from cell nuclei to detect recurrences.

### Five-Year Survival Rates:

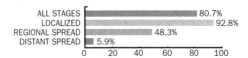

| | |
|---|---|
| ALL STAGES | 80.7% |
| LOCALIZED | 92.8% |
| REGIONAL SPREAD | 48.3% |
| DISTANT SPREAD | 5.9% |

0  20  40  60  80  100

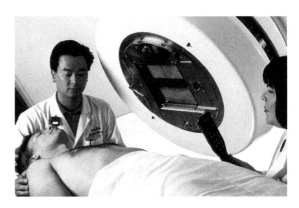

**HEALTH WORKERS position equipment for delivering radiation to a patient.**

## NON-HODGKIN'S LYMPHOMA

- **52,700 new cases to be diagnosed in the U.S. this year**
- **23,300 deaths expected**

**Risk Factors:** Because lowered immune system function raises susceptibility to this group of diseases, infectious agents that lower immunity, such as HIV, which causes AIDS, and HTLV-I, increase risk. Recipients of organ transplants are also at higher risk because of the immunosuppressive drugs they must take. Further possible dangers include occupational exposure to herbicides and perhaps other environmental chemicals.

**Warning Signs:** Enlarged lymph nodes; generalized itching; fever; night sweats; anemia; weight loss.

**Detection and Diagnosis:** Biopsy of affected lymph nodes. The grade, or characteristics of the proliferating cells, strongly influences the choice of therapy. X-rays of the lymphatic system, computed tomographic scans and ultrasonography can help determine how far the disease has spread.

**Treatment Now:** Non-Hodgkin's lymphoma includes about 10 different types of disease. Lymphoblastic and small noncleaved types are the most aggressive. Chromosome rearrangements associated with different forms of the diseases offer clues about how well or badly the cancer cells may respond to therapy.
Asymptomatic low-grade lymphomas may be treated with radiation or left untreated. Chemotherapy is now commonly used, because results with this approach have improved. Patients with higher-grade lymphomas are given chemotherapy and radiotherapy. Relapses are common and may be treated with high-dosage chemotherapy in combination with bone marrow transplants.
*Under study:* Various ways of improving the efficacy and safety of bone marrow transplantation; monoclonal antibodies directed at lymphoma cells.

### Five-Year Survival Rates:

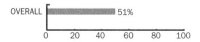

*In non-Hodgkin's lymphomas, grade is more important than tumor stage. People with low-grade tumors have a good chance of surviving longer than 10 years.*

**Controversies:** Researchers disagree about the classification and proper treatment of some uncommon types of non-Hodgkin's lymphomas.

## UTERINE CANCER

• **49,700 new cases to be diagnosed in the U.S. this year (15,700 for cervical, 34,000 for endometrial)**

• **10,900 deaths expected (4,900 from cervical, 6,000 from endometrial)**

**Risk Factors:** *For cervical cancer:* Sexual intercourse before age 18; many sexual partners (at least partly because of attendant risk of sexually transmitted papillomaviruses); cigarette smoking; low socioeconomic status. Mortality rate from cervical cancer is more than twice as high for black women as for white women.
*For endometrial cancer:* Exposure to estrogen, including estrogen replacement therapy not accompanied by progestin; tamoxifen treatment; early onset of menstruation; late menopause; never having been pregnant; other medical conditions, including diabetes, gallbladder disease, hypertension and obesity. The use of modern "combination" oral contraceptives appears to provide protection.

**Warning Signs:** Abnormal uterine bleeding. Pain occurs late in the course of the disease.

**Detection and Diagnosis:** Pap smear tests can find abnormal cells prefiguring cervical cancer. (One third of U.S. women do not undergo this test, however.) Pelvic exams are more effective at detecting endometrial cancer. Women at high risk should have an endometrial tissue sample evaluated at menopause.
*Under study:* Tests for mutations in genes regulating DNA repair may help warn of endometrial cancer.

**Treatment Now:** For cervical cancer, surgery or radiation, or both. Precancerous cells in the cervix may be eliminated by cryotherapy (use of extreme cold to kill cells), electrocoagulation (use of electricity) or local surgery. Endometrial cancer is treated by surgery, possibly with radiation and either hormone treatments or chemotherapy.

### Five-Year Survival Rates:

**For cervical cancer:**

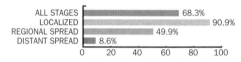

**For endometrial cancer:**

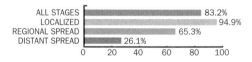

**Controversies:** Experts disagree over whether it may be reasonable to delay treatment of early-stage cervical cancer detected during pregnancy to improve the chances of survival of the fetus.

## MELANOMA OF THE SKIN

- **38,300 new cases to be diagnosed in the U.S. this year**
- **7,300 deaths expected**

*Melanoma accounts for three quarters of all deaths from skin cancer. The incidence has increased by 4 percent each year since 1973. (Basal cell and squamous cell skin cancers, which are not melanomas, account for more than 800,000 skin cancer cases in the U.S. annually but cause only 2,100 deaths because they are highly curable.)*

**Risk Factors:** Exposure to the sun, especially during childhood. Melanoma occurs most frequently in people who have fair skin that burns or freckles easily. Whites are 40 times more likely than blacks to develop melanoma.

**Warning Signs:** A change in the size, color, texture or shape of a mole or other darkly pigmented area; the appearance of a new, abnormal mole; spontaneous bleeding from a mole. Changes in other bumps or nodules in the skin are also suspect.

**Detection and Diagnosis:** Early detection is crucial. Adults should practice self-examination of the skin once a month and report to a physician any bleeding or sudden change in size or color involving a molelike growth, especially any that are asymmetric or have an irregular border. Biopsy may be needed to confirm diagnosis.

**Treatment Now:** Surgical removal of the melanoma.
*Under study:* Biological therapies, including interleukin-2 and interferon; therapeutic vaccines containing melanoma antigens, which are showing considerable promise.

### Five-Year Survival Rates:

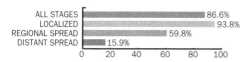

| | |
|---|---|
| ALL STAGES | 86.6% |
| LOCALIZED | 93.8% |
| REGIONAL SPREAD | 59.8% |
| DISTANT SPREAD | 15.9% |

0   20   40   60   80   100

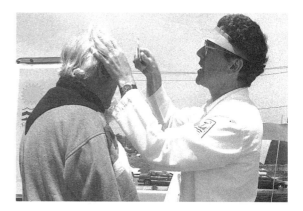

**SKIN CANCER CHECKUP for passersby in a beach community aims to find melanoma or other tumors.**

## KIDNEY CANCER

- **30,600 new cases to be diagnosed in the U.S. this year**
- **12,000 deaths expected**

**Risk Factors:** Males have twice the risk of females. Cigarette smokers have twice the risk of nonsmokers. Excess weight increases risk for some types of disease. Coke-oven workers and asbestos workers also have higher rates of kidney cancer.

**Warning Signs:** Blood in urine; lump in the area of the kidney; a dull ache or pain in the back or side. Occasionally, signs include high blood pressure or an abnormal number of red blood cells.

**Detection and diagnosis:** X-ray of kidneys, involving injected dyes; CT scans; magnetic resonance imaging scans; arteriograms; ultrasound exams. Biopsy needed to confirm diagnosis.
*Under study:* Mutations of the von Hippel-Lindau (VHL) gene in biopsy samples may indicate cancer.

**Treatment Now:** Removal of all or part of the affected kidney, usually with the adjoining adrenal gland. Radiotherapy and embolization, a procedure to block blood vessels, may be used to make symptoms less severe. Interleukin-2, a substance that plays a role in the immune system, is approved for use but can produce severe toxic side effects.
Because kidney cancer is often caught fairly early and sometimes progresses slowly, the

chances of surgical cure are frequently good. It is also one of the few cancers for which there are well-documented cases of spontaneous remission without therapy.

*Under study:* Biological therapeutic drugs, including interleukin-2 and interferon, for advanced kidney cancer; use of interleukin-2 along with immune system cells that have been grown and activated outside the body; biological therapy after surgery for early-stage kidney cancer; other new anticancer drugs.

**Five-Year Survival Rates:**

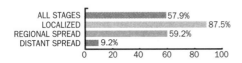

therapy of the central nervous system is used against ALL and may also be used against other types. Bone marrow transplants in combination with chemotherapy can treat chronic myelogenous leukemia (CML). Interferon therapy has also shown value.

*Under study:* New combinations of drugs and treatment regimens; biological agents; bone marrow transplantation for CLL, antisense therapy for CML.

**Five-Year Survival Rates:**

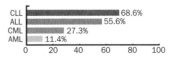

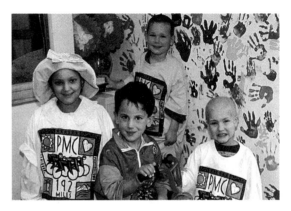

PATIENTS in a play area at the Dana-Farber Cancer Institute model T-shirts made for a fund-raising event.

## LEUKEMIA

- **27,600 new cases to be diagnosed in the U.S. this year**
- **21,000 deaths expected**

*Contrary to common belief, leukemia strikes many more adults than children. Acute lymphocytic leukemia (ALL) is the most common form among children; in adults the common types are acute myelogenous leukemia (AML) and chronic lymphocytic leukemia (CLL).*

**Risk Factors:** Certain genetic abnormalities, including Down's syndrome, Bloom syndrome and ataxia-telangiectasia; excessive exposure to ionizing radiation and some chemicals, such as benzene, found in lead-free gasoline; exposure to the virus HTLV-I.

**Warning Signs:** Fatigue, paleness, weight loss, repeated infections, ready bruising, nosebleeds and other bleeding. In children these signs can appear suddenly.

**Detection and Diagnosis:** Blood tests that look for abnormal white blood cells; bone marrow biopsy.

**Treatment Now:** Chemotherapy is the first-line treatment. Various combinations of anticancer drugs are employed in sequence, and transfusions of blood components and antibiotics are used to minimize the danger from infections. Radio-

## OVARIAN CANCER

- **26,700 new cases to be diagnosed in the U.S. this year**
- **14,800 deaths expected**

**Risk Factors:** Increasing age; never having been pregnant; family history of breast cancer or ovarian cancer; living in an industrial country (except Japan); an inherited mutated *BRCA1* or possibly *BRCA2* gene.

**Warning Signs:** Enlargement of the abdomen; rarely, abnormal vaginal bleeding. In women older than 40, vague digestive discomfort may also be indicative. Often, few symptoms appear.

**Detection and Diagnosis:** Periodic, thorough pelvic exams; transvaginal ultrasound; tests for a tumor marker substance (CA 125 antigen) in women suspected of having ovarian cancer. Biopsy is the definitive test, however. Women older than 40 should have a cancer-related physical checkup each year.

**Treatment Now:** Surgical removal of one or both ovaries, the uterus and the fallopian tubes is standard. In some very early tumors in young women, only the involved ovary will be removed. Radiation is also commonly employed, which may be administered by placing a radioactive liquid in the abdomen. Chemotherapy is sometimes used. Doctors measure blood levels of CA 125 and other substances to monitor responses to therapy.

*Under study:* The use of chemotherapeutic drugs put directly into the abdomen via a catheter. Gene therapy using the product of the *BRCA1* gene.

### Five-Year Survival Rates:

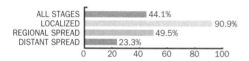

ALL STAGES 44.1%
LOCALIZED 90.9%
REGIONAL SPREAD 49.5%
DISTANT SPREAD 23.3%

0 20 40 60 80 100

**Controversies:** Testing for mutated *BRCA1* gene as an indicator of high risk. Physicians disagree over whether chemotherapy is valuable as an adjunct to surgery for early-stage disease.

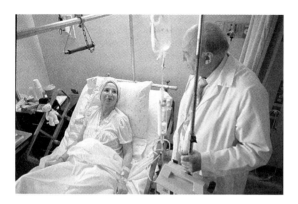

USE OF TAXOL has so far been approved for ovarian and breast cancer.

## PANCREATIC CANCER

- **26,300 new cases to be diagnosed in the U.S. this year**
- **27,800 deaths expected**

**Risk Factors:** Increasing age; cigarette smoking. Chronic pancreatitis, diabetes and cirrhosis may also be factors. Incidence is higher in countries with high-fat diets. The disease is also more common among blacks than whites, and the mortality rates have slightly risen among black women.

**Warning Signs:** Usually none until disease is advanced.

**Detection and Diagnosis:** Biopsy

*Under study:* The use of ultrasound imaging and CT scans for detecting cancers sooner.

**Treatment Now:** Tumors that are not small and confined to the pancreas are hard to treat.

Surgery, radiation and standard anticancer drugs can be used if the cancer has not metastasized, but usually diagnosis is too late for these approaches. To alleviate the pain of the disease, radiotherapy, surgical procedures to clear the bile ducts and nerve blocks can be effective.

*Under study:* Octreotide, a biological agent that has stabilized disease in a few patients. New surgical techniques that may improve quality of life; drugs that increase tumor sensitivity to radiation; various biological therapies and new anticancer agents.

### Five-Year Survival Rates:

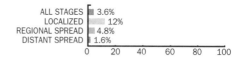

ALL STAGES 3.6%
LOCALIZED 12%
REGIONAL SPREAD 4.8%
DISTANT SPREAD 1.6%

0 20 40 60 80 100

*When the tumor is smaller than two centimeters and confined to the "head" of the pancreas—the end connected by a duct to the intestine—surgery offers a five-year survival rate of 20 percent.*

**Controversies:** The value of chemotherapy for many patients is questionable, but at least one regimen has prolonged survival without markedly impairing quality of life in carefully selected patients.

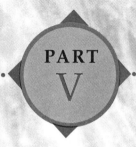

# THERAPIES OF THE FUTURE

**F**ascinating new approaches to treatment would combat cancers without the devastating side effects of many current therapies. Some capitalize on insights into how the immune system might be enlisted to destroy malignancies. Others are based on detailed knowledge of how tumors grow and spread.

# Immunotherapy for Cancer

*As knowledge about the immune system grows, scientists
are devising ways, using the body's own defenses, to attack cancer.*

• • •

Lloyd J. Old

Uring the past century, excitement has waxed and waned over the possibility that the extraordinary disease-fighting prowess of the immune system might be enlisted to destroy cancers. Today doubts have vanished, and countless investigators are working to translate the notion into potent new biological therapies.

Clinical support for the idea that the immune system might restrain the development of cancer emerged in the 1800s, when physicians noticed that tumors sometimes regressed in cancer patients who contracted bacterial infections. William B. Coley, a surgeon at Memorial Hospital in New York City from 1892 to 1936, dedicated his life to creating therapies based on this observation. He made deliberate attempts to infect cancer patients with bacteria and later devised a vaccine consisting of killed bacteria to prompt a tumor-killing response. These treatments—which we would now consider immunotherapies because they aimed to attack disease with the body's own defenses—brought about complete tumor regressions in some individuals. But they were not broadly accepted, because the results were unpredictable.

Early in this century other investigators also attempted to develop immune-based therapies, but none showed a convincing benefit. Still, the link between immunity and cancer remained firmly fixed in the minds of many people. During the 1960s and 1970s, for example, there was wide acceptance of the "immunosurveillance" model put forth by Lewis Thomas of New York University and MacFarlane Burnett of the Hall Institute in Melbourne, Australia. This theory held that the immune system constantly seeks out and destroys emerging cancer cells. Tumors, it proposed, arise when this policing mechanism fails. In the following years, however, accumulating evidence suggested that the immune system attacked only tumors caused by viral infections. Because such cancers account for a minority of all cases, the theory appeared flawed.

Recently, though, new insights have generated a resurgence of interest in immunotherapies for cancer. In particular, the science of immunology has undergone revolutionary changes. Researchers have discovered and isolated the cells and chemicals that enable the immune system to defend the body against attack and to prune away infected and damaged tissues. By studying these components, immunologists have gained a deep understanding of the workings of the normal immune system. And cancer immunologists have gained knowledge of mechanisms and molecules by which they may someday control cancer.

## Activating the Immune System

Today we would describe Coley's approach to cancer therapy as nonspecific: it strengthened the overall activity of the immune system instead of selectively arousing those elements most able to combat cancers. During the past decade, scientists have developed a range of other nonspecific immunotherapies. The strategy behind all these interventions has been likened to kicking the television set to make it work: give the immune system a good jolt, the thinking goes, and its capacity to rid the body of cancer cells may increase. Exactly which component, or combination of components, accounts for the killing remains unknown. Even so, the tactic has had some real success.

For instance, cancer occurring on the inner wall of the bladder—superficial bladder cancer—responds well to a vaccine, called Bacillus Calmette-Guérin, or BCG, used to combat tuberculosis. These mic-robes do not cause disease, because they evoke a strong immune response. Superficial bladder cancer typically recurs after surgery and, in its later phases, invades the bladder wall and beyond. But instilling BCG into the bladder by way of a catheter elicits a chronic inflammatory response—a prolonged activation of immune cells that fight invaders. Just how the inflammatory cells work is not understood in detail, but the end result is that the immune cells and the substances they secrete kill preexisting and developing cancer cells in the bladder wall. Consequently, patients who receive BCG postoperatively face a much lower risk of recurrence.

Although this vaccine illustrates the potential of nonspecific immunotherapies, it acts locally—provoking inflammation only in the bladder. Most cancers become lethal because they spread and give rise to tumors at distant sites. To eliminate those growths, immunotherapies must be capable of seeking out incipient tumors in all parts of the body. To accomplish this, many research oncologists turned in the 1970s and 1980s to molecules that the body produces in response to viral and bacterial infections; these molecules, now called cytokines, help to orchestrate the defense response. The cytokines include such proteins as interferons, interleukins and tumor necrosis factor (TNF). Investigators were initially very hopeful that cytokine therapy would be of great value. Extensive clinical testing

of this nonspecific approach, though, has dampened enthusiasm. Relatively few patients appear to benefit from cytokine therapy alone.

## Cancer Antigens

Cytokines may prove more valuable in combination with one another or with other treatments. Meanwhile, however, researchers have sought more specific ways to battle tumor cells. To single out cancer cells, an immunotherapy must be able to distinguish them from normal cells. One way the immune system can recognize differences among cells is by molecules, called antigens, that appear on the cell surface. Long ago scientists speculated that cancer cells might display molecules that signaled their abnormality. If such cancer-specific antigens were found, investigators could presumably devise means to make them more visible to the immune system. In other words, the antigens could be made to serve as targets for an immune attack—just as bacterial and viral antigens alert the body to disease-causing invaders.

The discovery of antibodies at the end of the 19th pressed into service as targets for antibody-based therapies. Many workers tried this approach and claimed to identify cancer-specific antigens. Unfortunately, none of these claims held up to careful scrutiny.

## The Era of Monoclonal Antibodies

The search for cancer antigens became easier in 1975, thanks to a discovery made by César Milstein and Georges J. F. Köhler of the University of Cambridge. These researchers demonstrated that antibody-producing cells could be made to survive indefinitely if they were fused with cancer cells. The technique, which earned Milstein and Köhler a Nobel Prize, enabled scientists to produce unlimited supplies of identical antibodies, or monoclonal antibodies, because any given antibody-producing cell produces only a single species of antibody. The method had a profound effect on cancer immunology for several reasons. First, it provided a powerful new method to search for cancer antigens. And second, workers could at last produce defined antibodies in sufficient amounts to put antibody-based therapies to the test.

Naturally, this spectacular technology gave rise to high expectations as well as to premature and unrealistic assertions about antibodies as "magic bullets." It was hoped that monoclonal antibodies

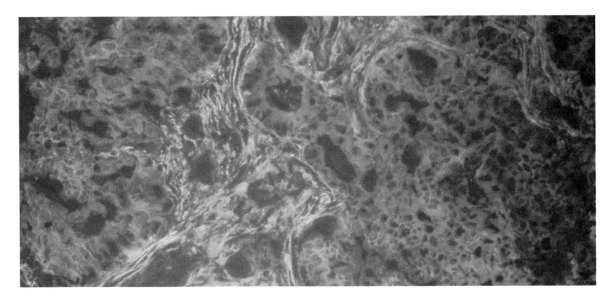

Figure 9.1 COLON CANCER SPECIMEN was stained using two monoclonal antibodies of different hues. Each antibody binds to distinct proteins on the surface of different cell populations. In this case, green marks cancer cells, and orange reveals the connective tissue (stroma). Because antibodies recognize specific cells, they can be used to find and selectively destroy tumor cells as well as the tissues that support and nourish such growths.

would home in on cancer cells (by recognizing specific antigens) and trigger an immune attack that destroyed the target cells but ignored normal cells lacking the cancer antigens. Many expected that these bullets could be made more deadly by loading them with toxic chemicals; the antibodies would carry the toxins directly to tumors, where the poisons would kill cancer cells. Excitement prompted industry and private investors to spend vast sums of money. But when the claims could not be substantiated as quickly as everyone hoped, opinion swung in the other direction, prompting many analysts and investors to declare that the technology had failed. The reality of the situation is far more positive. The concept remains sound, and slow, steady progress is being made in developing antibody therapies.

Monoclonal antibodies have revealed a large array of antigens that exist on human cancer cells. Regrettably, virtually all these antigens are also found on normal cells, which might therefore be damaged by an antibody-based therapy. This overlap, however, does not preclude their use as therapeutic targets for several reasons: the antigen in normal tissues may not be accessible to blood-borne antibodies; the cancer cells may express more antigen than normal cells do; and antibody-induced injury of normal cells may be reversible.

In addition to targeting cancer cells, antibodies can also be designed to act on other cell types and molecules necessary for tumor growth. For instance, antibodies can neutralize growth factors-chemicals needed by cancer cells and their blood supply—and thereby inhibit a tumor's expansion. And antibodies can target the stroma, the connective tissue between tumor cells (see Figure 9.1).

Without the stroma, which can make up 60 percent or more of a cancerous mass, a tumor cannot exceed a harmless, microscopic size. At the Memorial Sloan-Kettering Cancer Center in New York City, Wolfgang J. Rettig, Pilar Garin-Chesa and I have identified an antigen called FAP-alpha that is strongly expressed by stromal cells in a wide range of human cancers. This and other antigens that mark tumor stroma or tumor blood vessels have become attractive targets to researchers devising antibody-based therapies.

Today monoclonal antibodies are most often obtained from mice that have been immunized with human cancers. In clinical tests, human subjects generally mount an immune reaction that inactivates the injected mouse-derived molecules. Scientists have therefore begun to construct human therapeutic antibodies that should evade immune recognition. In the meantime, workers are disguising

## Landmarks in the History of Tumor Immunotherapy

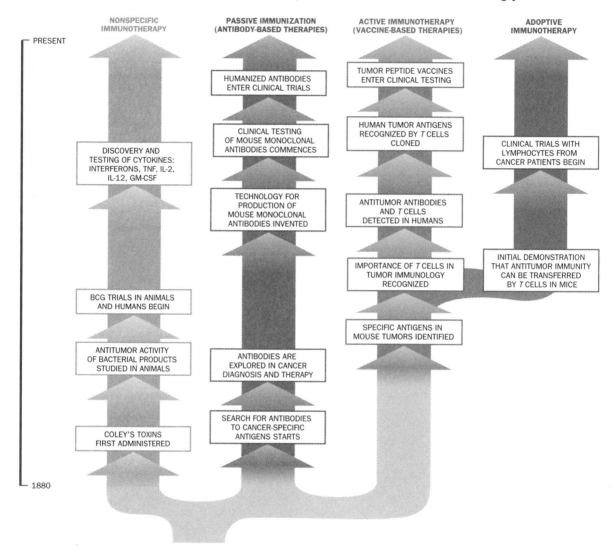

the murine antibodies, refashioning them into something more resembling human antibodies. They do so by replacing all the nonessential structures in the mouse antibody with the corresponding human parts. This trick, called humanization, has yielded antibodies that in initial clinical tests have sneaked past the human immune system. Antibody engineers are also refining other characteristics of the humanized molecules to make them better able to bind to antigens and penetrate tumors.

### Testing Antibodies in the Clinic

Once a target antigen is identified and an antibody construct selected, antibody engineers must decide what kind of toxic message they wish to deliver to a tumor. Here lie two distinct approaches. One ex-

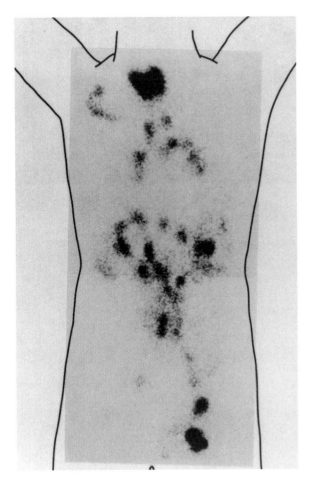

Figure 9.2 COLON CANCER METASTASES in the abdomen and elsewhere are dark on this scan because they have absorbed and concentrated the monoclonal antibody A33, labeled with a radioactive isotope. Normal intestinal cells also take up A33 but do not retain it. (Thyroid takes up released radioactive isotope.) It is this selective accumulation of monoclonal antibodies in tumors that raises hopes of targeted therapies having fewer side effects than conventional chemotherapies.

ploits the ability of antibodies themselves to destroy cancer cells. The other, as envisioned from the start, uses antibodies as vehicles to carry a toxic agent— be it a chemotherapeutic agent or a radioactive compound, a plant or a bacterial toxin—to a tumor site. Many new antigenic targets and antibody constructs have emerged—so many, in fact, that they cannot all be tested in the clinic.

One criterion for deciding which antibody to test as a therapy is the likelihood that it will be taken up by a tumor in significantly greater amounts than by normal tissues. To see if an antibody meets this requirement, it is tagged with a radioactive isotope of iodine ($^{131}$I), injected into human volunteers and followed in the body using imaging techniques. For a more accurate assessment of the antibody's accumulation in the tumor, a biopsy is taken. Because none of the antigenic targets studied so far exist exclusively on tumors, imaging studies are also critical for discerning how much antibody attaches to normal tissues. Antibodies showing favorable characteristics in these studies are the best candidates for therapeutic trials.

To develop even one antibody-based therapy requires tremendous effort and time, which explains why translating good ideas into useful therapies can proceed much more slowly than anyone would like. Consider the ongoing studies of a mouse monoclonal antibody called A33, carried out by Sydney Welt and our group at Memorial Sloan-Kettering. This antibody detects an antigen that is expressed by normal cells in the intestine and by virtually all colon cancers (see Figure 9.2). Clinical studies using A33 labeled with a trace of radioactive isotope showed substantial uptake in colon cancers. Up to one hundredth of a percent of the injected antibody accumulated in the tumor mass. Moreover, the antibody was able to penetrate the core of the tumor.

These favorable results justified taking A33 to the next step: clinical trials with a therapeutic aim. We loaded the antibody with much higher doses of radioisotope, designed to irradiate and destroy cancer cells, and asked two key questions: Can enough antibody reach the tumor, and what effect will the isotope-carrying antibody have on normal cells in the gastrointestinal tract? Because the human subjects in the trial mounted an immune response that neutralized the mouse-made A33, only a single injection of the molecule could be given. (Follow-up injections would be useless because the immune system would recognize and eliminate the antibody before it had the opportunity to come near a tumor.) Even with such limited dosing, the tumors in some patients shrank.

Most important and surprising, we observed that the antibody caused no toxicity in the gut even though it accumulated there. We believe the gut cells are not harmed by the antibody because they rapidly excrete it. In contrast, the tumor cells retain it. A humanized version of A33 has been developed and is now being tested in the clinic. To give some idea of the timescale involved in these studies, the antigen was identified in 1982; the first clinical study started in 1988; the therapeutic trials com-

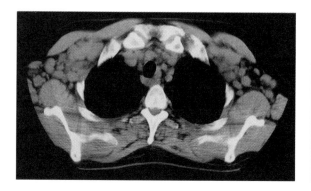 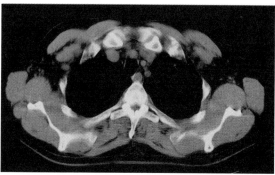

Figure 9.3   COMPUTED TOMOGRAPHIC SCANS show a cross section of a 41-year-old man's upper torso before and after treatment for lymphoma with CD20 antibody-based radioimmunotherapy. The large black circles are the lungs. Despite earlier chemotherapy regiments, the patient had extensive disease, marked by many enlarged lymph nodes (*left*). After a single CD20 treatment (*right*), however, all disease disappeared. The patient continues to be in complete remission two years later.

menced in 1991; and the first patients were injected with the humanized antibody in 1995.

Perhaps the major success in the field to date comes from studies of an antibody that binds to an antigen on both healthy *B* cells—immune cells that, once activated, manufacture antibodies—and on lymphomas of *B* cell origin. Stuart F. Schlossmann of the Dana-Farber Cancer Institute in Boston originally described this antigen target, called CD20, and it has since been studied by a number of groups, including that of Mark S. Kaminski of the University of Michigan and Oliver W. Press of the University of Washington School of Medicine. The results are quite exciting (see Figure 9.3). The antibody alone can bring about tumor regressions, and when it is combined with $^{131}$I, these regressions are substantial and prolonged. Equally important, the therapy produces few side effects. Thus, we know that even if an antigen is expressed on normal cells, it can, as had been hoped, still serve in some cases as a useful target for therapy.

As with most experimental therapies for cancer, those based on antibodies are generally tested in patients who have advanced forms of the disease. But these therapies may be far more effective if used sooner. Gert Riethmüller of the University of Munich has in fact studied the effect of a monoclonal antibody called 17.1A in patients who have colorectal cancer in fairly early (basically localized) stages. He started antibody therapy in these individuals immediately after they had their visible tumors removed by surgery. Despite surgery, some patients remain at high risk because of residual cancer cells. But in Riethmüller's study, the antibody-treated patients had a significantly lower recurrence rate. Treating the cancer cells left behind after surgery—or those beginning to spread to some other site—makes much sense, and all forms of immunotherapy will undoubtedly focus on this goal in the future.

## The Promise of Vaccines

In the antibody-based therapies we have been discussing, the injected antibody derives from an animal; in the future, it may be made in a test tube. Either way, the treatment is considered passive immunotherapy: the immune molecules are given to patients, who do not produce them on their own. A vaccine, on the other hand, is deemed active immunotherapy because it rouses an immune response in the individual who needs protection.

Efforts to treat cancer with vaccines date back to the very origins of immunology. Over the years, doctors have vaccinated many hundreds of cancer patients with malignant cells—either the patients' own cells or those taken from another patient— usually irradiated to prevent further growth. Although occasional responses were observed, this early vaccination strategy suffered from major deficiencies. Most significant, it offered no way to monitor the vaccine's effect on the immune system. When vaccines against infectious diseases such as polio-myelitis were developed, their impact could

# Tumor-Killing Agents Delivered by Antibodies

Acting alone, antibodies bind to antigens on the surface of cancer cells. In doing so, they mark these cells for destruction by other immune components or cause them to self-destruct. Antibodies can similarly target and attack the blood vessels feeding a tumor or the connective tissues (or stroma) supporting it. And antibodies can neutralize or block the action of growth factors—chemicals that a tumor needs to grow. In addition, antibodies are used as guided missiles of sorts. They can deliver an array of damaging compounds (some of which are listed below) to tumor sites.

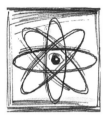

**Radioactive isotopes,** such as iodine 131 or yttrium 99, kill cancer cells by damaging their DNA.

**Other toxins** travel to a tumor site by way of antibodies. One well-studied example is ricin, which is made from castor beans; it inhibits protein synthesis and thwarts tumor growth. Toxic products from bacteria and other microorganisms also stall cancer cells in experiments. And many other highly tumoricidal drugs too toxic to be used alone-including CC-1065, calicheamicin and maytansinoids— may be effective if targeted by an antibody.

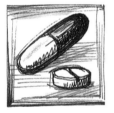

**Chemotherapeutic drugs** often reach tumors in larger, and so more lethal, doses when delivered by an antibody.

**Enzymes** that can convert innocuous "prodrugs" into cell killers will home to tumors when attached to antibodies. Because the enzymes activate the prodrugs only at tumor sites, healthy tissues in the body remain unharmed.

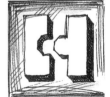

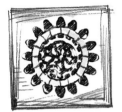

**Genetic drugs** come in several forms. So-called antisense DNA molecules block the production of proteins needed by cancer cells. Other gene constructs give rise to proteins that kill tumor cells; the genes can be linked to antibodies directly or packaged into viral particles engineered to have targeting antibody on their surface.

**Inflammatory molecules,** which include tumor necrosis factor (TNF) and other messenger molecules of the immune system as well as certain microbial products, can bring about an inflammatory reaction that destroys tissues at the tumor site.

**Immune cells** guided by antibodies, such as genetically engineered *T* cells, can prompt tumor cell dissolution, or lysis.

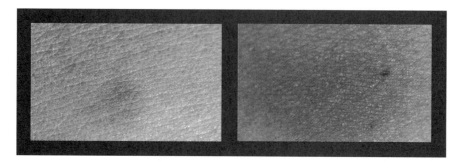

Figure 9.4   SKIN TESTS offer one way to tell if a patient's immune system recognizes peptide antigens expressed by tumor cells. If so, irritation in the form of a so-called delayed hypersensitivity reaction appears on the skin. The initial skin reaction (*left*) in this melanoma patient became more pronounced after the injection of an immune-boosting cytokine, GM-CSF (*right*). This response resembles the tuberculin reaction that follows a tuberculosis vaccination and can be used to monitor whether a vaccine is stimulating a patient's immune system as intended.

be readily detected by looking for the specific antibodies they elicited. But until recently, scientists had no comparable information about cancer antigens and the immune response they provoke. Without such knowledge, investigators had no hope of understanding why the treatment seemed to work in some cases but not in others. Steady progress over the past several decades has now brought us to a point where we can place the development of cancer vaccines on a firm scientific basis.

The modern vaccine story starts in the 1940s and 1950s with a fundamental discovery of tumor immunology. Scientists found that when chemicals or viruses induced tumors in mice, the tumors bore antigens that could immunize other mice of the same strain against transplants of the tumors. Subsequent studies showed that immune system cells known as *T* lymphocytes taken from immunized animals could transfer immunity against tumors to healthy animals of the same strain. And workers devised techniques to show that the *T* cells from the immunized mice could kill tumor cells grown in test tubes as well. In contrast, antibodies elicited by the tumor cells generally failed to transfer immunity or kill tumor cells.

As a next step, we needed to see if comparable immune reactions would take place in humans. For ethical and practical reasons, we could not apply the same approach used in the animal studies described above. And so the focus was on immune reactions that could be extensively analyzed in test tubes. Our group chose to examine melanoma cells, in part because they can be easily grown in the laboratory. Over a 10-year period, we studied a large number of melanoma patients, seeking evidence of antibodies or *T* cells in these patients that reacted with their own melanoma cells. We found that a small proportion did mount a specific immune response against their own tumor cells. And we also formed the impression that these patients followed a more favorable clinical course.

The next challenge was to isolate the tumor antigens recognized in this system so that they might be tested in a vaccine. Thierry Boon and his colleagues at the Ludwig Institute for Cancer Research in Brussels developed a method to do just that for *T* cell recognized antigens [see "Teaching the Immune System to Fight Cancer," by Thierry Boon; SCIENTIFIC AMERICAN, March 1993]. This technique has revealed two main categories of tumor antigens that evoke a *T* cell response in melanoma patients. The first includes antigens called MAGE, BAGE and GAGE that are produced by tumor cells but not by any normal cells outside the testes. The other category of antigens, including tyrosinase and Melan A, are so-called differentiation antigens; they are made by both melanoma cells and melanocytes, normal cells from which the tumor cells arise.

*T* cells do not "see" the whole protein antigen on the cancer cell, but only pieces of it, termed peptides (see Figure 9.4). When the tumor cell processes the protein, it presents these peptides on the cell surface in conjunction with so-called histocompatibility antigens. Scientists are now creating a rapidly growing list of protein and peptide tumor antigens, identified using the method developed by Boon and his group to clone tumor antigens. All

# Categories of Cancer Vaccines

Cancer vaccines are intended to induce *T* cells or other components of the immune system to recognize and vigorously attack malignant tissue.

**Whole cancer cells**    Inactivated cancer cells and their extracts can jump-start the immune system. Cancer cells engineered to secrete cytokines, such as IL-2 or GM-CSF, similarly heighten antitumor immunity. Cells designed to express co-stimulatory molecules, such as B-7, enhance the ability of *T* cells to recognize tumor cells.

**Peptides**    Tumor peptides, fragments of tumor proteins recognized by *T* cells, are injected alone or with immune-boosting adjuvants.

**Proteins**    Antigen-presenting cells take up injected tumor proteins and break them down into a range of peptide fragments recognized by *T* cells.

**Dendritic cells**    These antigen-presenting cells are isolated from the blood, exposed to tumor peptides or engineered to produce tumor proteins and then reinjected.

**Gangliosides**    Humans can produce antibodies to these molecules, such as GM2, found on the surface of tumor cells. Clinical studies have shown that melanoma patients with GM2 antibodies.

**Heat-shock proteins**    These cellular constituents ordinarily bind peptides. Injecting heat-shock proteins isolated from tumors rouses antitumor immunity in mice.

**Viral and bacterial vectors**    Genes coding for tumor antigens are incorporated into viral or bacterial genomes. When injected, these altered infectious agents draw immunity against themselves and the encoded antigens.

**Nucleic acids**    DNA and RNA coding for tumor antigens prompt normal cells to begin producing these antigens.

these molecules are prime candidates for use as vaccines. Even newer techniques promise to extend the list of possible vaccines.

Another source of information about potential tumor antigens comes from the avalanche of discoveries concerning genetic changes in cancer cells. Any alteration in a cancer cell that can be recognized by the immune system is grist for the cancer immunologist's mill. Among the most attractive targets for vaccines are abnormal proteins that are made when genetic mutations turn normal genes into cancer-promoting versions. A long list of cancer-related genes—known as oncogenes and tumor suppressor genes—is now being compiled (see Chapter 1,

## Tactics Tumors Use to Evade Immune Attack

### ALTERING THEIR CHARACTERISTICS

Under attack by the immune system, tumor cells generate variants lacking those features that mark them for destruction by T cells, other killer cells and antibodies. The process, called immunoselection, can lead to tumor cells that do not have tumor antigens or major histocompatibility antigens, which present tumor antigens to immune cells. Tumor cells can also lack co-stimulatory molecules, which activate T cells, and signaling molecules needed to respond to cytokines, such as gamma-interferon, that promote tumor cell killing by immune mechanisms.

### SUPPRESSING THE IMMUNE SYSTEM

Tumor cells can effect changes in the host that diminish or abrogate an effective immune response against them. Specific immunosuppression occurs when tumor cells deliver inappropriate or ineffective signals to T cells, reducing their number or ability to respond. Nonspecific immunosuppression is caused by other tumor cell products, such as TGF-beta, or by cancer drugs or irradiation.

### HIDING FROM THE IMMUNE RESPONSE

Immune reactions are less effective or absent in several sites in the body, such as the brain, and so tumors there avoid immune attacks. Also, a dense tumor stroma consisting of connective tissues can shield tumor cells from immune recognition and destruction.

### EXPLOITING THE IMMUNE SYSTEM'S IGNORANCE

Tumor cells may grow without eliciting any immune response. But an effective immune response can be generated by immunizing against tumor antigens—indicating that the potential for immune attack is not always activated.

### OUTPACING THE IMMUNE RESPONSE

Tumor cells can simply proliferate so quickly that the immune response is not fast enough to keep their growth in check.

---

"How Cancer Arises"). And, of course, human cancers caused by viruses, such as cervical cancer, are prime targets for vaccine-based therapies.

As is the case with monoclonal antibody therapies, there are now more vaccine-based therapies than anyone can test in patients. And, although medicine's vast experience with vaccines against infectious diseases will help guide cancer vaccinologists, much uncharted territory lies ahead. Whole-cancer-cell vaccines, whether genetically engineered or not, will probably give way to vaccines that contain defined tumor antigens. Moreover, because peptide vaccines are easy to synthesize, they are taking center stage in clinical trials. In early tests, some tumor regressions have already been noted. Some cancer immunologists theorize

that whole proteins will be more effective as vaccines because they can provoke the immune system with a range of different peptides. Scientists eagerly await large supplies of pure tumor antigens to test the idea.

Yet another approach to immunotherapy is under study. Known as adoptive immunotherapy, it involves stimulating T cells by exposing them to tumor cells or antigens in the laboratory and then injecting expanded populations of the treated cells into patients. In contrast to the studies in inbred mice, where T cells from one mouse can be given to any other mouse of the same strain, T cells from one person would generally be rejected by another person. For this reason, patients serve as both donor and recipient of their own T cells. Steven A.

Rosenberg of the National Cancer Institute spearheaded the clinical testing of this approach, and efforts continue to make this therapy more effective and less time-consuming and expensive.

Adoptive immunotherapy may have its greatest value in treating viral infections and tumors in patients whose immune systems have been weakened by disease and therapy. For instance, before leukemia patients receive bone marrow transplants, they receive massive doses of chemotherapy and radiation to destroy all leukemia cells. This leaves the individuals immunosuppressed and vulnerable to infections, such as cytomegalovirus infection (CMV). But there are now indications that an injection of CMV-specific *T* cells can reduce the risk of CMV infection in such transplant patients. In addition, dramatic regressions of virus-related lymphomas arising in transplant patients can be brought about by simply injecting lymphocytes from normal donors. Because these immune cells are spared the effects of the immunosuppressive drugs, they retain their ability to combat the lymphoma cells.

## The Hurdles Ahead

Despite the great hope of immunotherapy, a dark cloud hangs over all our attempts to control cancer by immune mechanisms. Cancer cells are masters of deceit and disguise—veritable Houdinis that can readily alter themselves to evade immunologic recognition and attack (see the box "Tactics Tumors Use to Evade Immune Attack").

Because the race is between immune control and escape, the best strategies to combat cancer will need to attack it on several fronts. Opportunities being explored include constructing vaccines that combine a variety of antigens (called polyvalent vaccines); testing how well antibody- and vaccine-based approaches work together; and combining nonspecific and specific immunotherapies and other cancer therapies.

Other potential obstacles need our attention as well. As noted with antibodies, it is conceivable that cancer vaccines may injure normal cells to some degree. There are a number of disease states, called autoimmune diseases, that arise when the immune system turns against normal tissues in the body. Examples include rheumatoid arthritis, multiple sclerosis and certain forms of kidney disease. It may turn out that some modest degree of autoimmunity is the price we pay for a successful cancer vaccine.

Given the long history of tumor immunology—marked by recurrent cycles of high expectations and disappointments—we need to exert considerable caution in making any predictions. But many promising opportunities wait to be studied, and they give us reason to expect that powerful immunologic therapies will one day become a reality.

Perhaps these therapies will yield cures—the universal objective of cancer researchers, health care providers and, of course, patients. A more achievable aim, though, may be developing therapies that can change the nature of cancer from a progressive and lethal disease to one that can be controlled throughout a long life. That result would be less than ideal, but it could make a world of difference for many afflicted with tumors not readily treatable today.

# New Molecular Targets for Cancer Therapy

*Investigators are exploiting the characteristic molecular abnormalities of cancers in new approaches to treatment.*

• • •

Allen Oliff, Jackson B. Gibbs and Frank McCormick

Before the 1980s, scientists had little understanding of how tumor cells acquire their lethal properties of uncontrolled growth and spread. Researchers identified beneficial new drugs primarily by exposing tumor cells to various compounds and seeing whether the chemicals halted cell division. Or they injected cancer-stricken animals with a compound and assessed shrinkage of the tumors. Unfortunately, many agents that attacked cancer cells also damaged healthy tissue, such as normal bone marrow and intestinal cells and thus gave (and continue to give) rise to unpleasant and sometimes dangerous side effects.

Recently the molecular defects that transform normal cells into malignant ones have begun to come clear (see Chapter 1, "How Cancer Arises"). Many of these defects consist of mutations in key classes of genes that are responsible in some way for the reproduction, or growth, of cells. Those mutations alter the quantity or behavior of the proteins encoded by growth-regulating genes and, in so doing, disrupt functions that control cell division. Knowledge of mutant genes is enabling pharmaceutical researchers to design new drugs that will specifically act on disrupted genes or their proteins. Such drugs, it is hoped, will restore normalcy to malignant cells or short of that, kill the cells without significantly harming healthy ones. Although most of these drugs are only beginning to be tested, preliminary results encourage us about the prospects of controlling cancer at its molecular level (see Figure 10.1).

The defects targeted by molecular therapy are found in three classes of genes. The first class, known as oncogenes, stimulates cell progression through the cell cycle—the sequence of events in which a cell gets larger, replicates its DNA and divides, passing a complete set of genes to each daughter cell. Members of the second class restrict such growth; they are referred to as tumor suppressor genes. Genes in the third group govern the replication and repair of DNA. Most tumors possess mutations in one or more of these gene categories.

We will discuss each category and explain the biochemistry involved. We will also indicate how an anticancer drug could be delivered to cells and how it might stop cancerous development. Finally, we will briefly discuss the therapeutic prospects.

Although virtually any known genetic defect can suggest ideas for therapy, we will focus on treatments that have a reasonable chance of becoming available within the next 10 years.

## Oncogenes: Activating Cancer

Oncogenes are mutant versions of normal genes (sometimes called proto-oncogenes) that drive cell growth. The differences between oncogenes and normal genes can be subtle. The mutant protein that an oncogene ultimately creates may differ from the healthy version by a single amino acid. Yet that one alteration can radically change the protein's function.

The most common cancer-causing mutation of this kind occurs in the *ras* gene. Approximately 20 to 30 percent of all human cancers harbor an abnormal *ras* gene. The protein encoded by the *ras* gene (the Ras protein) ordinarily behaves as a relay switch within the signal pathway that tells the cell to divide: in response to stimuli transmitted to it from outside the cell, it activates the rest of the signaling pathway.

In the absence of outside prompts, the Ras protein would normally remain in the "off" state. The mutated Ras protein, however, behaves like a switch stuck in the "on" position. It continuously misinforms the cell, instructing it to divide when it should not. These observations suggest that a compound able to block the action of the mutant Ras protein could be an effective anticancer agent. (Such blocking compounds are called antagonists.) But how can the mutant Ras protein be inactivated?

One potential answer became evident when researchers began to understand how the Ras protein is made (see Figure 10.2). Newly formed Ras molecules are functionally immature. These precursor versions must undergo several biochemical modifications to become mature, active versions. Then the Ras proteins attach to the inner surface of the cell's outer membrane, where they can interact with other cellular proteins and stimulate cell growth.

**Figure 10.1  TREATING CANCER at the molecular level includes repairing faulty DNA, shutting down key growth** proteins and increasing tumor cells' sensitivity to conventional therapies, such as radiation.

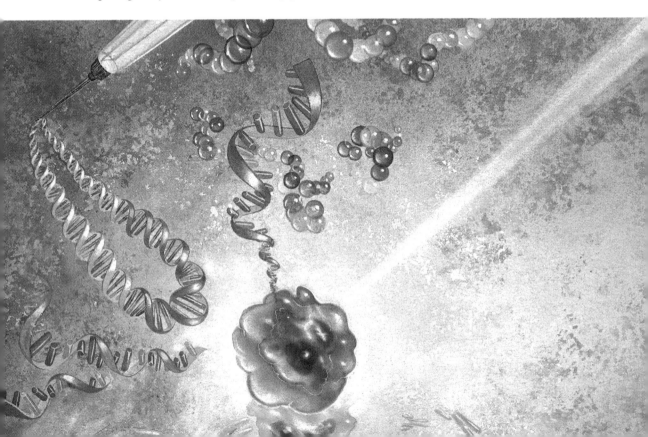

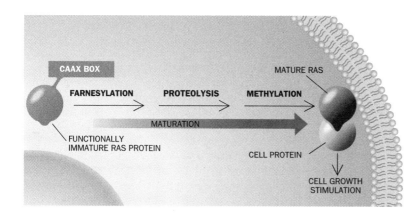

Figure 10.2 RAS PROTEIN begins as an inactive precursor. Maturation takes place in three steps at the so-called CAAX box. Once modified, Ras can interact with other proteins and stimulate cell growth. Drugs that block the farnesylation reaction and thus prevent the Ras protein from becoming active could stop tumor cells from dividing.

The changes take place at one end of the Ras precursor, where enzymes act on a region called the CAAX box. The modification happens in three steps, the most critical being the first, called the farnesylation step. In this step, 15 carbon atoms are added to the precursor. A specific enzyme, termed farnesyl transferase, catalyzes the reaction.

One strategy for blocking Ras protein activity has been to inhibit this enzyme and thus stop the modification. Investigators have created several such inhibitors. In cell cultures, these inhibitors block the maturation of the Ras protein and reverse the cancerous transformation induced by mutant *ras* genes. Tests on animals have provided encouraging results as well. They showed that farnesyl transferase inhibitors prevented the formation of new tumors by abnormal Ras proteins. They also induced the regression of existing cancers of this type.

Fortunately, farnesyl transferase inhibitors seem quite specific. The drugs do not affect normal cells or cells transformed by other oncogenes. Their specificity suggests that side effects might be minimal. Indeed, many of these inhibitors given at high doses—enough to eliminate preexisting tumors—have exhibited virtually no toxicity to normal tissues in animals.

Another set of oncogenes ripe for exploitation as anticancer targets are those that encode enzymes termed protein kinases. (Some cancers in which mutated kinase genes have been found include chronic myelogenous leukemia, breast cancer and bladder cancer.) In normal cells, protein kinases help to regulate many important processes. Some of these activities include sending signals between the cell membrane and the nucleus, initiating a cell's progress through the cell cycle, and controlling various metabolic functions of the cell. Protein kinases control these processes by activating other proteins in response to particular stimuli.

Kinases can lead to cancer in a couple of ways. Overproduction, caused by mutations in the control regions of their genes, is one. Compared with normal cells, tumor cells frequently manufacture extremely high levels of one or another kinase. The vast quantities keep the cells dividing when they should stop. A commonly overproduced kinase in cancerous tissue is the receptor for epidermal growth factor (EGF).

Kinases can also contribute to cancer if their structure is abnormal. Many tumor cells possess protein kinases that because of some structural defect are permanently turned on. They therefore carry out reactions that inappropriately stimulate cells to divide. Some examples of kinases that behave abnormally in certain human cancers are the Abl, the Src and the cyclin-dependent kinases (see Figure 10.3).

Obviously, an inhibitor of one or more of these kinases might be an effective anticancer agent. The challenge is finding a drug that can distinguish one kinase from another. Many of the nearly 1,000 protein kinases in mammalian cells have highly similar structures, particularly in their biochemically active regions. Hence, an inhibitor of any single protein kinase might disrupt the activity of other, unrelated kinases crucial for normal cellular functions.

Despite this concern, pharmaceutical researchers have synthesized and tested a series of kinase inhibitors over the past few years. Most target the kinases themselves, but others attack at the genetic level (preventing the kinases from being made). For instance, in the so-called antisense approach, snippets of genetic material interfere with the tumor cell's messenger RNA, thus impeding the formation of proteins. Messenger RNA molecules are essentially mobile copies of genes and are the physical templates from which cells construct the proteins encoded by genes [see "The New Genetic Medicines," by Jack S. Cohen and Michael E. Hogan; SCIENTIFIC AMERICAN, December 1994].

Remarkably, kinase inhibitors can be quite selective. In the test tube, some find their intended target 1,000 times more frequently than they do unrelated kinases. More important are findings from whole cells in culture. They show that several of these compounds inhibit the growth of cancer cells that possess mutated protein kinase genes. Even more encouraging, some of these agents have also been shown to block the growth of tumor cells in animals—a sign that they might work in the human body. These drugs offer hope that some protein kinase antagonists will be available in the next few years to treat human cancers.

## Tumor Suppressor Genes

The second main category of genes responsible for cancer includes those that, when working properly, suppress the development of malignancies. Many cancers result from the loss or malfunction of the key regulatory proteins that these genes encode. The two primary tumor suppressor proteins are the pRB and the p53 proteins.

The pRB protein (which draws its name from "retinoblastoma," the type of tumor in which its gene, called *RB*, was first identified) helps to regulate the cell cycle. In particular, its active form serves as a brake to DNA replication. In about 40 percent of human cancers, mutations in the *RB* gene render its protein inactive. As a result, the cells divide nonstop.

Another profoundly important regulatory molecule is the p53 protein. Often called the guardian of the genome, it prevents replication of damaged DNA in normal cells and promotes suicide, or apoptosis, of cells with abnormal DNA (see Figure 10.4).

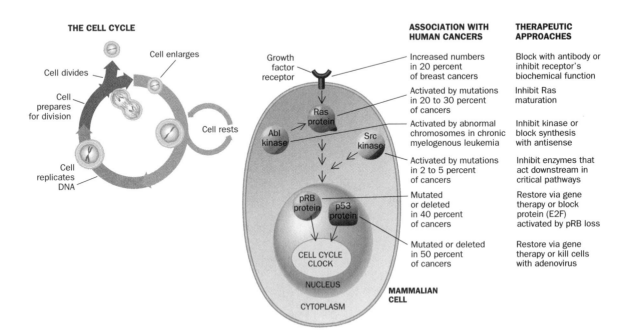

Figure 10.3 SIGNALING PATHWAY in a mammalian cell (*right*) includes many components that, when altered in quantity or structure, can lead to cancerous growth. Among these components are growth factor receptors, Ras protein and the kinase enzymes that aid their function, such as Abl and Src. Perturbations of pRB and p53 can foster cancer development as well. The changes cause the cell cycle (*left*) to go out of control.

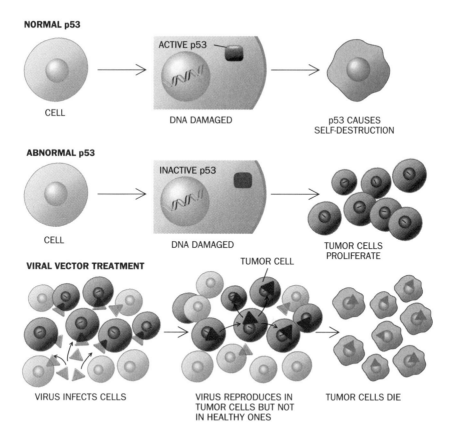

**NORMAL p53**

CELL → DNA DAMAGED (ACTIVE p53) → p53 CAUSES SELF-DESTRUCTION

**ABNORMAL p53**

CELL → DNA DAMAGED (INACTIVE p53) → TUMOR CELLS PROLIFERATE

**VIRAL VECTOR TREATMENT**

TUMOR CELL

VIRUS INFECTS CELLS → VIRUS REPRODUCES IN TUMOR CELLS BUT NOT IN HEALTHY ONES → TUMOR CELLS DIE

Figure 10.4 p53 PROTEIN instructs a cell to kill itself if the DNA is damaged by, say, drugs or radiation. But if p53 is abnormal, it may not stop a cell with bad DNA from replicating. One way of treating tumor cells is through viruses genetically engineered so that they reproduce in cells with abnormal p53 but not in healthy cells. In principle, the virus would move unchecked only through tumor cells, killing them.

Faulty p53 molecules allow cells carrying damaged DNA to survive when they would normally die and to replicate when they would normally stop; the disturbed cells pass any existing mutations down to their progeny, which then have the opportunity to accumulate any additional mutations they might need to form lethal tumors. In most human cancers, the *p53* gene appears defective.

What therapeutic strategies can tackle malfunctioning *RB* and *p53* genes? Several general approaches have been considered. Conceptually, the most straightforward is to replace the defective gene with its normal counterpart. Referred to as gene therapy, the process has appeared encouraging in cell culture experiments: normal *RB* or *p53* genes introduced into tumor cells blocked the growth of those cells. Investigators are now devising protocols for clinical trials. They hope to introduce normal *p53* genes into tumor cells in humans.

Researchers are actively exploring various methods for delivering genes into tumor cells. Weakened viruses could carry a normal gene and deliver it only to tumor cells (see the box "Sending in Tumor-Targeting Viruses"). This viral vector approach, however, is still new and faces a number of difficulties, not the least of which could be a preemptive strike by the immune system. It might kill the viruses before they have had a chance to reach tumor cells.

## Regulating the Gene Products

Given the hurdles facing gene therapy, many oncologists studying tumor suppressors are instead

# Sending in Tumor-Targeting Viruses

Perhaps the most promising way to reach tumor cells is through viruses. In gene therapy, weakened viruses can act as couriers that deliver normal genes into cells. The best of these viruses in terms of its potential ability to deliver therapeutic genes to cancer cells is the adenovirus. Adenoviruses contain DNA (some viruses, such as retroviruses, have only RNA). If a gene useful for therapy is spliced into the viral DNA, the virus will deliver the needed gene into any cell it invades. The virus will do no harm as long as its own genes that confer virulence are removed when the new gene is inserted.

Adenoviruses can also kill tumor cells specifically. When a virus enters a normal cell, so-called p53 proteins respond by instructing the infected cell to stop making DNA, thus preventing the virus from replicating. An adenovirus protein can bind directly to p53 and thereby disable it. Then the virus can use the cell's machinery to replicate itself.

The adenovirus can be genetically altered in such a way that it assumes command of tumor cells only, not healthy ones. Specifically, the p53-binding protein of the adenovirus can be made so that it can no longer bind to p53. As a result, the virus cannot shut down p53. Therefore, it can only replicate in cells that lack normal p53—namely, many varieties of tumor cells. Indeed, studies have shown that such modified viruses replicate efficiently in tumor cells and proceed to make identical viral progeny. In theory, these viruses can then go on to infect adjacent tumor cells and thus spread throughout a cancer. All the cells in a tumor may be infected and killed in this way.

Viral vector approaches are in their infancy, and several technical hurdles still need to be tackled. Perhaps the most critical is ensuring that a sufficient fraction of the tumor cells are infected and that any newly introduced gene produces enough of its normal protein to stop the tumor cells and improve and sustain the patient's health. There might also be immunologic reactions to the viral vector protein—for instance, the immune system may attack and neutralize the virus before it reaches its target. The ultimate utility of this approach in cancer therapy may depend on the extent to which the immune response can be controlled during treatment. One kind of attenuated adenovirus is now moving toward clinical trials and should begin preliminary testing in patients within the next couple of years. Investigators are also exploring other delivery methods, using alternative kinds of viruses (for example, retroviruses) and lipids that would not provoke an immunologic response.

exploring a more traditional approach. It entails assessing the chain of events stemming from genetic defects in a cell and then developing drugs that treat one of those events. For example, in healthy cells the pRB protein blocks the activity of another protein (called E2F), which, when free, promotes the synthesis of DNA. Loss of the pRB protein therefore leads to uncontrolled E2F action and rampant cell proliferation. It follows, then, that drugs able to inhibit E2F could halt the expansion of tumors arising from the loss of pRB protein.

Currently the effects that such an inhibitor would have on normal cells are hard to predict. But recent experiments, such as studies of mice in which the *E2F* genes have been specifically "knocked out," now make it feasible to model the potential side effects. By extrapolating these results to humans, we can anticipate the harmful effects of these drugs—and perhaps find ways to evade them—years before clinical trials.

Researchers know the biochemical pathway regulated by the *RB* gene, but they cannot say the same for that of *p53*. We do not know precisely the molecular chain of events that stem from the loss of the *p53* gene. As a result, most of the potential drug targets downstream of p53 have not yet been identified.

A curious feature of p53 protein inactivation, though, presents an opportunity. Some test-tube experiments suggest that normal p53 function can be restored with small molecules, which, when attached to a mutant, inactive p53 protein, would reactivate it. If a similar feat can be achieved in tumor cells, we would expect the malignant cells to stop growing or even die, because one function of p53 is to make abnormal cells self-destruct. The technical feasibility of this approach is challenging, but the potential value is immense, given the number of cancers that have bad *p53* genes. Efforts are under way in many laboratories to explore this strategy.

### Genes That Check DNA Repair

The third major category of genes that could be molecular targets encompasses those that help to check and maintain the integrity of DNA, which is often damaged during replication. Without these mechanisms, the chances that a damaged gene will be repaired fall drastically, and the likelihood rises that the damage will ultimately be transmitted to the cell's progeny as a permanent mutation. Indeed, tumor cells frequently have defects in their DNA repair processes. For instance, 10 to 20 percent of human colon cancers appear to have mutations in genes that ordinarily help to repair DNA (the *MLH1, MSH2, PMS1* and *PMS2* genes).

Other genes indirectly participate in DNA repair; in fact, mutations of these genes are much more common. Among these genes are ones encoding "checkpoint" proteins, which monitor a cell's progress through the cell cycle and prevent the next stage from occurring if earlier stages have not been traversed successfully—for instance, if DNA has not been copied accurately. The most notable checkpoint proteins are ATM and, once again, the versatile p53. Tumor cells that lack normal *ATM* or *p53* genes are missing these checking mechanisms. Any damaged DNA is rushed through the replication process, increasing the frequency of random mutations in the daughter cells.

As with the mutated tumor suppressor genes, gene therapy might be used to replace missing or damaged genes that encode DNA-repairing or related proteins. A more radical approach may be to allow some tumors to mutate themselves to death. Tumor cells that increase their mutation rate pay a price: many mutations are lethal and lead to the death of the daughter cells. The tumor can afford to lose many of its progeny as long as a few

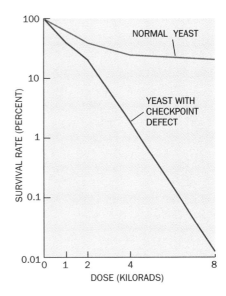

**Figure 10.5 DNA CHECKPOINT DEFECT increases yeast cells' sensitivity to radiation. An eight-kilorad dose leaves many healthy yeast alive but virtually wipes out those that cannot properly check their DNA repair mechanisms. Such a finding suggests that damaging checkpoint DNA in tumor cells could make them more vulnerable to conventional cancer therapy.**

of the acquired mutations enhance the survival of at least some of the tumor's descendants. But if too many mutations are generated, then none of the tumor's daughter cells may be viable.

One way of nudging cancer cells to produce daughter cells that cannot survive is to inhibit several checkpoint mechanisms simultaneously. Ordinary yeast cells exposed to DNA-damaging x-rays die only after high radiation doses. But if one of its checkpoint genes is mutated, the yeast become more sensitive to radiation (see Figure 10.5). In fact, if two or more checkpoint genes mutate at the same time, the cells become hypersensitive to radiation. Even low doses kill them.

Based on these observations, oncologists are designing drug-screening assays to identify agents that inhibit checkpoint proteins. These drugs could act on tumor cells possessing a known defect in a checkpoint gene (a mutant *p53* gene, say). With many such defects, the cancerous cells should readily die or at least succumb easily to other treatments. Several compounds have shown some promise in cell cultures, although clinical trials

# Molecular Approaches in Cancer Therapy

| CANCER FEATURE | MOLECULAR TARGETS | THERAPEUTICS |
| --- | --- | --- |
| Oncogene activation leading to excessive Ras protein or kinase activity | Ras proteins | Farnesyl transferase inhibitors: L-744, 832; SCH 44342; BZA-5B |
| | Abl, EGF receptor, Erb-B2 and Src kinases | Tyrosine kinase inhibitors: tyrphostins (RG 13 022); lavendustins (AG 957); quinazolines (PD 153 035) Antisense inhibitors |
| | PKC-$\alpha$, Raf and cyclin-dependent kinases | Serine/threonine kinase inhibitors: olomoucine; staurosporine; butyrolactone Antisense inhibitors |
| Loss of tumor suppressor genes | *APC, AT, DCC, RB* and *p53* genes | Gene therapy to restore normal suppressor gene function Antisense agents to block E2F synthesis |
| Abnormal DNA repair mechanisms | DNA mismatch repair enzymes: MSH2; MLH1; PMS1; PMS2 | Gene therapy to restore normal enzyme activity Checkpoint inhibitors to promote susceptibility to DNA-damaging agents |
| Lack of senescence (cell aging) in tumor cells | Telomerase | Telomerase inhibitors |
| Angiogenesis | FGF, VEGF growth factors Integrin receptors | TNP-470; suramin $\alpha_v\beta_3$, $\alpha_v\beta_5$ antagonists |
| Metastases | Metalloproteases Collagenases | Protease inhibitors Collagenase inhibitors |

probably will not begin until after the turn of the century.

Besides targets involved in cell growth, molecular therapies can also aim for other important molecules; some of these therapies could be available in the next four years. For example, various proteins keep cells in one place in the body; with this knowledge, workers have discovered drugs, such as protease inhibitors, that might prevent cancer cells from metastasizing, or spreading, throughout the body (see Chapter 2, "How Cancer Spreads"). Other drugs will try to disable telomerase, the enzyme that rebuilds the ends of replicating chromosomes and in so doing enables cancer cells to remain immortal under conditions when other cells would die. Compounds, such as one called TNP-470, might choke off the formation of new blood vessels (angiogenesis) that nourish tumors (see Chapter 11, "Fighting Cancer by Attacking Its Blood Supply").

Although the targets for drugs outlined here represent some of the most exciting advances in cancer biology over the past decade, a word of caution is appropriate concerning the speed with which these findings can be converted into practical therapeutics. The new medicines based on these modern observations must overcome many of the same obstacles standard chemotherapies have had to surmount. Not only must they locate their cancerous targets, but they also must find a way to penetrate into malignant cells in sufficient numbers to be effective. Solid tumors pose a multitude of barriers to drug delivery; not much blood flows deep inside tumors, and some drugs might not easily perfuse out of blood vessels that feed tumors and then find their way into the cancerous mass itself [see "Barriers to Drug Delivery in Solid Tumors," by Rakesh K. Jain; SCIENTIFIC AMERICAN, July 1994]. And of course, there are the issues of toxicity, side effects and the emergence of drug resistance in the tumor cells.

The latest methods of pharmaceutical science can be used to foster drug discovery. These methods include recombinant genetics to produce compounds, genetically engineered animals to serve as model systems, high-volume robotic screening of compounds, combinatorial chemistry techniques and computer-assisted design of drugs. Even when these techniques are employed, most anticancer agents take at least 10 years to become available, as measured from the time the molecular target is first identified until novel drugs for that target can be discovered, developed and approved for use.

First, two to three years of molecular, genetic and cell biological studies are needed to confirm that a target is indeed critical to the development of human cancers. Thereafter biochemical screening assays to find promising compounds require a year or two. Once a good lead is discovered, medicinal chemists modify the drug to optimize its potency, specificity and pharmacological properties. These efforts will typically consume another three to five years and demand the synthesis of several hundred to several thousand related compounds. Once in the clinic, traditional three-phase evaluations of the agents can take another three to five years or longer to determine unequivocally their safety, efficacy and proper doses.

This timetable for drug discovery and development presents a sobering reality for basic cancer researchers and clinical oncologists alike. Nevertheless, several molecularly targeted, mechanism-based cancer therapeutics are far along in the drug-development pipeline. Antisense drugs that inhibit protein kinases began clinical trials earlier this year. The farnesyl transferase inhibitors and several other kinase inhibitors should begin clinical trials in the next two to four years. The gene therapy approaches intended to replace mutated genes with their normal counterparts are further away, at least a decade.

Besides its laser-beam accuracy, the molecularly targeted approach may have another favorable characteristic. For reasons that are not yet clear, tumor cells with multiple molecular defects seem to respond even when only one of these defects is treated. Therefore, a patient may not need to take several drugs simultaneously to get some benefit.

Although formidable obstacles stand in the way, the next generation of cancer therapies holds the potential of being more effective and less toxic. With a plethora of targets to aim for, chances are good that a number of compounds will provide powerful new ammunition in the war on cancer.

# Fighting Cancer by Attacking Its Blood Supply

*By interfering with the expanding network of blood vessels
in tumors, researchers hope to cut off the underlying support system.*

• • •

Judah Folkman

The tiny blood vessels known as capillaries extend into virtually all the tissues of the body, replenishing nutrients and carrying off waste products. Under most conditions, capillaries do not increase in size or number, because the endothelial cells that line these narrow tubes do not divide. But occasionally—for example, during menstruation or when tissue is damaged—these vessels begin to grow rapidly. This proliferation of new capillaries, called angiogenesis or neovascularization, is typically short-lived, "turning off" after one or two weeks.

But neovascularization can also occur under abnormal conditions: tumor cells can "turn on" angiogenesis (see Figure 11.1). As new blood vessels bring in fresh nutrients and proteins known as growth factors, the tumor mass can expand. In fact, neovascularization appears to be one of the crucial steps in a tumor's transition from a small, harmless cluster of mutated cells to a large, malignant growth, capable of spreading to other organs throughout the body. Tumor cells are usually unable to stimulate angiogenesis when they first arise in healthy tissue; unless the deranged cells become vascularized, the mass will not become larger than about the size

of a pea. Thus, if researchers can determine how mutated cells trigger angiogenesis and, more important for patients, how to interrupt the process, they will have a powerful new anticancer therapy at their disposal. Furthermore, because antiangiogenic drugs stop new growth but do not attack healthy vessels, they should in theory do no harm to blood vessels serving normal tissues. (Angiogenesis inhibitors can stop menstruation or delay wound healing, however.)

Research into the importance of angiogenesis to the progression of cancer has been a vital area of laboratory investigation for several decades—I wrote an early article on the subject in the mid-1970s [see "The Vascularization of Tumors," by Judah Folkman; SCIENTIFIC AMERICAN, May 1976]. But only in the past seven years has research moved out of the laboratory and into the clinic. In 1989 the first clinical trial of an anti-angiogenic agent—interferon alpha—began for the treatment of life-threatening hemangioma (a noncancerous blood vessel tumor found primarily in infants).

By 1992 the first antiangiogenic drug for cancer patients, TNP-470 (a synthetic analogue of the substance fumagillin), entered clinical trials. The first studies were restricted to a few kinds of tumors, but the Food and Drug Administration now allows physicians to administer TNP-470 in clinical trials for a wide variety of cancers in humans. In the past four years, at least seven other angiogenesis inhibitors have entered clinical trials for the treatment of advanced cancer, and one of these compounds is also being tested in patients with abnormal blood vessel growth in the eyes.

The effort to explore the practical applications of antiangiogenic compounds reflects years of work by many researchers—unfortunately too numerous to list in this short space. For example, during the past several years, scientists have identified at least 14 different proteins found in the body that can trigger blood vessel growth and several others that can halt it. Most recently, researchers have discovered that one of these natural angiogenesis inhibitors is normally under the control of the tumor suppressor gene *p53*, which has been implicated in various cancers. With such clues, cancer researchers continue to refine their understanding of angiogenesis in tumor growth and of ways to block it.

## Angiogenesis Is Required for Spread

As with most aspects of cancer progression, angiogenesis distorts a normal biological process—in this case, regulation of blood vessel growth. Capillary blood vessels, each thinner than a hair, are arranged so that almost every healthy cell in the body can live directly on the surface of a capillary. If a healthy cell becomes cancerous and begins dividing rapidly, the resulting daughter cells accumulate in a microscopic mass. As the cells pile up, they find themselves farther and farther from the nearest capillary. When a few million such cells have accumulated, the small tumor—often called an in situ carcinoma—stops expanding and reaches a steady state, in which the number of dying cells counterbalances the number of proliferating cells. This restriction in size is caused in part by the lack of readily available nutrients, protein growth factors and oxygen. These minuscule carcinomas can be detected if they are on the skin or cervix, but in the breast, lung or colon, they may go unrecognized for several years. Regrettably, we do not yet

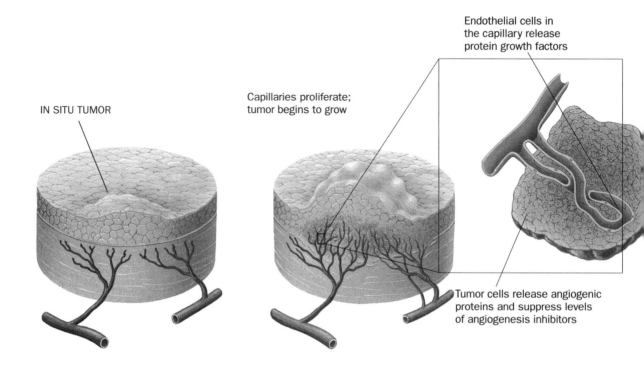

Endothelial cells in the capillary release protein growth factors

Capillaries proliferate; tumor begins to grow

IN SITU TUMOR

Tumor cells release angiogenic proteins and suppress levels of angiogenesis inhibitors

have the technology to detect most small in situ tumors in internal organs until after the tissue has been removed and examined under a microscope.

After many months or even years in this steady state, an in situ tumor may abruptly induce new capillary growth and start to invade surrounding tissue. The tumor calls into service naturally occurring proteins that promote neovascularization. The mutated tumor cells might themselves produce high levels of such proteins; alternatively, they can mobilize angiogenic proteins found in nearby tissue, or they may prompt other types of cells, such as macrophages, to release angiogenic proteins.

Yet even after employing these mechanisms, malignant cells may still fail to trigger angiogenesis. Recent discoveries by Noel Bouck's group at Northwestern University and in Douglas Hanahan's laboratory at the University of California at San Francisco suggest that certain tumor cells make two types of protein: one kind stimulates angiogenesis, and the other inhibits it. The balance between them determines whether the tumor can switch on angiogenesis. And experiments indicate that the ability to turn on angiogenesis most likely depends on a decrease in the production of those proteins that inhibit the process. So, in effect, angiogenic cancer cells release the natural brakes on the spread of new capillaries—once a tumor becomes angiogenic, it tends to stay that way.

Once neovascularization occurs, hundreds of new capillaries converge on the tiny tumor; each vessel soon has a thick coat of rapidly dividing tumor cells. Some of these cells are not angiogenic but are nonetheless sustained by capillaries recruited by neighboring cells. Now the tumor can expand rapidly—in a matter of months, the mass may reach one cubic centimeter in size and contain around one billion tumor cells.

Further promoting the progress of the disease, the newly dividing endothelial cells release at least six different proteins that can stimulate the proliferation or motility of tumor cells. For example, in breast cancer, the capillary endothelial cells recruited to the tumor produce the protein interleukin-6, which can increase the probability that breast cancer cells will leave the tumor, migrate into the bloodstream and

umor continues to expand, eventually spreading to other organs

After treatment with antiangiogenic drugs, tumor diminishes in size

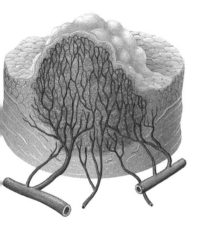
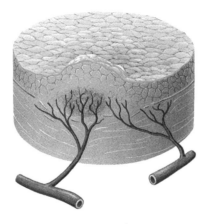

Figure 11.1 ANGIOGENESIS, or neovascularization, involves the proliferation of new blood vessels. The process transforms a small, usually harmless cluster of abnormal cells (known as an in situ tumor) into a large mass that can spread to other organs. Drugs that aim to interfere with angiogenesis—for example, by halting the action of angiogenic proteins—can reduce the size of tumors and potentially maintain them in a dormant state.

spread to other organs—in other words, metasta-size. Some of the metastases contain cells that are already angiogenic and thus will grow rapidly. Other metastases, however, contain mainly nonangiogenic cells and may lie dormant for years, becoming angiogenic long after the original tumor has been treated or removed (see Figure 11.2).

When a tumor has advanced to this stage, it often causes readily identifiable symptoms. Blood appearing between menstrual periods or in the urine, stool or sputum indicates that angiogenesis has taken place in the cervix, bladder, colon or lung, respectively. By the time a breast cancer can be seen on a mammogram, the tumor has already undergone vascularization. The bloody abdominal fluid seen with ovarian cancer, the bone pain of prostate cancer, the swelling around brain tumors and the obstruction of the intestinal tract common in colon cancer all result from angiogenic tumors. Biologically active molecules released by the expanding tumor can cause additional symptoms, such as weight loss and formation of blood clots.

## Shrinking Tumors

At present, patients diagnosed with any form of cancer typically rely on surgery or radiation to remove or eradicate the original tumor and on follow-up radiation or chemotherapy, or both, to try to eliminate any remaining cancerous cells in the body. Antiangiogenic therapy, in contrast to many other therapeutic approaches, does not aim to destroy tumors. Instead, by limiting their blood supply, it attempts to shrink tumors and prevent them from growing. Antiangiogenic drugs stop new vessels from forming around a tumor and break up the existing network of abnormal capillaries that feeds the cancerous mass. Currently, in addition to the angiogenesis inhibitors that are in clinical trials, many potential inhibitors are under study in university laboratories and in some 30 pharmaceutical and biotechnology companies around the world.

In particular, two of the compounds being looked at are very potent angiogenesis inhibitors, suggesting that they eventually will be quite useful for treating cancer patients. David A. Cheresh and his colleagues at the Scripps Institute discovered the first of these substances: a protein that interferes with another molecule known as an integrin, which is found in large quantities on the surface of growing endothelial cells. If the integrin (named $alpha_v beta_3$) is blocked, the proliferating endothelial cells die.

The second of these promising compounds, the protein angiostatin, was discovered in mouse urine by Michael S. O'Reilly in my laboratory at Children's Hospital Medical Center in Boston. Angiostatin is among the most potent of the known angiogenesis inhibitors. In animals, it can stop nearly all blood vessel growth in a large tumor or in its metas-

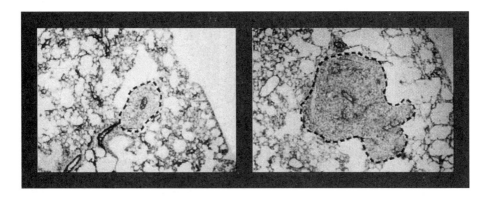

**Figure 11.2 METASTASES** can grow when levels of naturally circulating angiogenesis inhibitors, such as the protein angiostatin, fall. Angiostatin released by a large tumor in a mouse initially kept in check small metastases in the animal's lung (*left*). When researchers removed the original tumor, circulating angiostatin dropped off, allowing the metastases to expand (*right*) as blood vessels (*red*) proliferate. A similar pattern occasionally occurs in humans: after removal of one tumor, new metastases may appear, but primary tumors should be removed and follow-up chemotherapy can prevent the growth of metastases.

tases. Human prostate, colon and breast cancers that have been implanted in mice and allowed to grow to 1 percent of the animals' body weight can be reduced to a microscopic size and held in a dormant state for as long as angiostatin is administered. Furthermore, angiostatin is very specific, halting only the multiplication of endothelial cells and not of other cells or of normally quiescent endothelial cells. This specificity has powerful benefits: researchers have not detected in animals any toxic side effects of the drug. In addition, resistance to angiostatin does not appear to develop in animals.

Angiostatin is actually a fragment of the larger protein plasminogen, which is not antiangiogenic itself. Indeed, several angiogenesis inhibitor proteins exist as internal fragments of larger proteins (for instance, another inhibitor is a fragment of the protein prolactin), suggesting that normal angiogenesis inhibitors may be, in a sense, stored within larger proteins. Thus, when the body needs to stop normal angiogenesis—after wound healing or ovulation—these natural inhibitors may be available for immediate use by simply breaking down the larger proteins.

## Offering Treatment

Laboratory studies as well as ongoing clinical trials of angiogenesis inhibitors provide important guidelines for how these drugs may eventually be used in cancer patients, if they receive approval from the FDA. For example, when angiogenesis inhibitors are first introduced into clinical practice, they will most likely be used in combination with current conventional therapy. Beverly A. Teicher of the Dana-Farber Cancer Institute in Boston has shown in animals that combinations of angiogenesis inhibitors and chemotherapeutic agents are more effective than either therapy alone. In one instance, 42 percent of the animals were cured by a combination of treatments but not by either drug alone.

A possible explanation for the apparent synergism between these two therapies is that the two types of cells in a tumor—the endothelial cells and the tumor cells—respond differently to therapy. For example, endothelial cells have a low or virtually undetectable mutation rate as compared with that of tumor cells and thus do not usually become drug-resistant. In addition, every 10 to 100 new tumor cells require at least one new endothelial cell. (One gram of tumor contains approximately 20 million endothelial cells and 100 million to one bil-

lion tumor cells.) Therefore, when an angiogenesis inhibitor halts the growth of one endothelial cell, the effect on tumor cells may be amplified.

Angiogenesis inhibitors have also been studied in conjunction with radiation therapy. Oncologists and radiologists initially debated whether radiation therapy would be enhanced by coupling it with antiangiogenic drugs. But Teicher recently found that treatment of mouse tumors with angiogenesis inhibitors did increase the effectiveness of radiation therapy. Several antiangiogenic drugs, including TNP-470 and minocycline (a relative of the antibiotic tetracycline), are being examined in conjunction with radiation therapy in animals.

After the completion of conventional chemotherapy or radiation therapy, angiogenesis inhibitors might be used as a long-term treatment against cancer. If the cancer has metastasized, antiangiogenic therapy may be needed indefinitely. In other situations, antiangiogenic drugs may be given for a brief period, perhaps before surgical removal of a large tumor. Antiangiogenic treatment could possibly be administered intermittently, even for a few months or years, to maintain a tumor's dormancy. Fortunately, the general lack of drug resistance developed against these compounds as well as their low toxicity makes them amenable to extended use.

## Future Directions

Although scientists have been investigating angiogenesis for more than two decades, many questions remain about the process, how it is regulated and how it can be controlled therapeutically. For instance, no one understands why some tumors, particularly in the cervix, undergo neovascularization much earlier than others. And antiangiogenic drugs now in development face the traditional uncertainties of all clinical trials: unforeseen side effects could surface, or a drug might be ineffective in humans despite its efficacy in mice.

In addition, as with any new drug, there are potential economic hurdles to overcome. Many of the angiogenesis inhibitors are newly discovered proteins or other types of molecules. Chemists must now figure out how to make these compounds on a large scale. This process can be expensive, but experience suggests that prices should fall with time.

Despite the obstacles, antiangiogenic substances offer the promise of an additional anticancer therapy

# Angiogenesis Inhibitors in Clinical Trials

Although no antiangiogenic drugs have been approved for use in cancer patients, many are now in clinical trials.

| DRUG | POSSIBLE MECHANISM OF ACTION | CURRENT STATUS |
|------|------------------------------|----------------|
| CAI | Inhibits influx of calcium into cells, suppressing proliferation of endothelial cells | Phases I and II |
| CM101 | Induces inflammation in tumors, destroying growing capillaries | Phase I |
| Interferon alpha | Decreases production of the angiogenic protein FGF (made by tumor cells) | Phase III (hemangiomas in infants) |
| Interleukin-12 | Increases production of an angiogenic inhibitor called inducible protein 10 | Phase I |
| Marimastat | Inhibits the enzymes that cells employ when migrating through tissue | Phases II and III |
| Pentosan polysulfate | Blocks action of growth factors on endothelial cells | Phase III |
| Platelet factor 4 | Inhibits proliferation of endothelial cells | Phases I and II |
| Thalidomide | Exact mechanism unknown | Phases I and II |
| TNP-470 (AGM-1470) | Selectively inhibits proliferation and migration of endothelial cells | Phases I and II |

Phase I: Small trials to evaluate toxicity and determine maximum safe dose
Phase II: Small trials for signs of efficacy
Phase III: Large trials that compare new therapy with best available treatment

for our current armamentarium. Angiogenesis inhibitors may turn out to have significant benefits because they are not as likely to induce resistance and because they generally have fewer side effects. These agents may also be used to treat other diseases characterized by abnormal angiogenesis. Among these other conditions are diabetic retinopathy, macular degeneration and neovascular glaucoma—all diseases of the eye in which abnormal vessels proliferate and destroy vision. In addition, psoriasis, arthritis, hemangioma and other benign tumors may be susceptible to treatment with angiogenesis inhibitors. Clearly, then, antiangiogenic drugs have exciting potential as therapies for a number of serious conditions—in addition to cancer.

# PART
## VI

# LIVING WITH CANCER

There are ways to cope successfully with the physical, psychological and practical challenges of the disease. Resources are available to patients who know where to look. Even pain can usually be controlled—if caregivers award the problem the attention it deserves.

# Cancer's Psychological Challenges

*Cancer patients today have many options for easing distress.*
*These interventions may not prolong life, but they can improve its quality.*

• • •

Jimmie C. Holland

Until the second half of this century, "cancer equals death" was so pervasive a belief that physicians usually withheld the diagnosis from the patient and informed only the family. Families, in turn, often hid the fact that a member had the disease, as if it were something to be ashamed of. Today the stigma associated with cancer has largely vanished in the United States. Patients receive abundant information about their illness and are free to discuss available treatments with doctors and others.

These changes can be traced to the 1950s, when chemotherapeutic agents were successfully used, often in combination with surgery and radiation, to treat several types of cancer, notably acute leukemia and Hodgkin's disease in children and young adults. Those who first benefited from these advances sometimes exhibited "survivor guilt"—similar to that suffered by Holocaust survivors—as they struggled to understand why they had been spared when so many others had not. Such feelings are much less common today, when there are eight million cancer survivors in the United States alone.

Partly as a result of the women's and consumer-rights movements in the 1960s, cancer patients began to demand more information about their diagnosis and medical options. In the mid-1970s Betty Ford and Happy Rockefeller, both wives of nationally prominent politicians, pushed the issue farther out of the closet by disclosing their own struggles with breast cancer. Still, change has come slowly. In the 1970s, when I began to explore the psychological responses of patients to cancer, one oncologist warned me that I could talk to his patients only if I did not mention the disease itself.

A few years after that incident, the Memorial Sloan-Kettering Cancer Center in New York City created a psychiatry service, which was charged with conducting research and training young psychiatrists and psychologists in the new area of psycho-oncology. Our work focuses on two major issues: first, the psychological impact of cancer on the patient, the family and caregivers; second, the influence of psychological and behavioral factors on cancer risk and survival.

## Assessing Quality of Life

More specifically, we have asked such questions as: What are the common responses to cancer? Which ones are normal, and which are abnormal, reflecting a degree of distress that could interfere with a person's ability to follow a treatment plan? What is the prevalence of psychological problems warranting therapy? Do particular emotional reactions affect the course of illness, either adversely or positively? Finally, what interventions and coping methods can reduce distress?

One major goal of psycho-oncology has been developing ways to measure a patient's overall ability to function. By responding to detailed questionnaires, patients can quantify how they are functioning physically, psychologically, socially, sexually and at work, as compared to when they were well.

These methods are now applied widely to determine how a given treatment affects quality of life. In fact, the Food and Drug Administration recommends that quality of life be included as a secondary criterion, after survival rates, in assessments of most new cancer treatments. The result is that researchers can calculate a figure called quality-adjusted life years, or QALYS. This figure provides a more accurate picture of the potential benefits and adverse effects of a treatment—such as chemotherapy for women with recurrent breast cancer—than survival rates alone.

The psychological impact of cancer can obviously be devastating. The word still evokes fears of death, disfigurement, physical dependence and inability to protect those whom one holds dear. The immediate response of someone diagnosed with the illness is usually disbelief and shock. The person may think, "This can't be happening to me; they made a mistake in the slides." Next comes a phase of acute distress, turmoil and depression, which may include preoccupation with disease and death, anxiety, loss of appetite, insomnia, poor concentration and inability to carry out normal routines.

Ideally, after a week or two patients begin to feel all is not lost and to pursue a plan for treatment. Over the next weeks and months, they slowly learn to cope with the overwhelming reality of illness. The way people adjust to cancer over the long run has much to do with their prior ability to face life's problems and crises. Some cope with the challenges of the disease relatively calmly and constructively, whereas others—particularly those with preexisting psychological difficulties—may go into an emotional tailspin.

Anxiety attacks, insomnia, poor concentration, anorexia and a loss of interest in normal activities and even of the desire to continue living—all are signs of serious distress that should be addressed by a mental health worker if they persist several weeks beyond the initial diagnosis. People also need professional assistance if their responses interfere with medical care. Many people need such help. In a recent study done at three cancer centers, 47 percent of those diagnosed with cancer had a level of distress equivalent to that seen in a true psychiatric disorder. By far the most common problems were anxiety, depression or a combination of the two.

Sometimes troubling emotions are triggered by medications with mood-altering side effects, such as steroids and pain medicines. Identifying the source of distress is important so that the proper intervention can be prescribed. If medications are not at fault, psychotherapy or other forms of counseling may be effective, although antidepressants are often needed as well. Many patients are so afraid of addiction that they eschew drugs, whether antidepressants or painkillers, and needlessly endure severe psychic or physical pain (see Chapter 14, "Controlling the Pain of Cancer"). Those inclined toward stoicism must realize that reducing their suffering can make more bearable not only their own life but the lives of their loved ones as well.

Over the past two decades, communication between patients and physicians about psychological issues has improved. More patients ask that consideration be given to the "human side" of their care. Most doctors, for their part, have come to realize that how they convey bad news and otherwise relate to patients can have a profound effect on patients' morale and thus on their response to treatment. Caregivers are also increasingly taught to pay greater attention to patients' subjective assessments of their condition, including pain or psychological reactions.

Yet doctors may still have difficulty determining when a patient's normal feelings of sadness and anxiety have become so severe that they demand therapeutic intervention. One obstacle is that many patients avoid discussing their feelings because they do not want to be perceived as "weak" or "whiny." Doctors with little training in psychology or psychiatry may also avoid questioning patients about their emotional state—perhaps because they feel incompetent to explore this area, or they fear opening up a psychological "Pandora's box," or they think that the patient might be offended.

The result is a "don't ask, don't tell" situation in which psychological distress remains hidden—and therefore untreated. This is especially true of sexual problems, which both patient and doctor are often too embarrassed to mention. Yet patients are entitled to help; they can do themselves a favor by overcoming their reticence and raising their concerns with a doctor who fails to bring up the topic. Physicians can then either counsel patients directly or refer them to someone more qualified. Many hospitals now have psychiatrists or psychologists specializing in the care of cancer patients, and those that do not should be prepared to refer patients to appropriate therapists.

## Mind-Body Links

There has been enormous interest lately—on the part of both the medical community and the lay public—in the mind's effect on health. This interest has stemmed in part from intriguing findings linking various psychological states to changes in the endocrine and immune systems. Although no one knows yet to what degree such interactions apply to cancer, the findings have nonetheless led some advisers to promulgate rather simplistic psychological schemes for combating cancer.

Many articles, books and counselors exhort patients to "think positively" and to "fight" the illness. Patients have also been encouraged to visualize their immune cells attacking the cancer cells. The physician and philosopher Lewis Thomas, who died of a rare form of cancer in 1995, once told me that given the complexity of the immune system, he would not know which of his cells to encourage to fight.

Envisioning oneself as a warrior battling the cancer "dragon" can help those who previously faced life's problems that way. For those whose style is less assertive, the fighting model is not constructive. These individuals are often intimidated by their families and others who suggest, incorrectly, that an insufficiently aggressive attitude may hasten death. In truth, no single style of coping on the part of the patient has proved any better than all the others.

Moreover, large, well-controlled studies do not support the widespread belief that emotional factors—whether grief precipitated by a specific trauma or simply a gloomy or anxious predisposition—lead to cancer or accelerate its spread. This unfounded assertion has led some cancer patients to say they have been victimized twice—once by the disease and again by being blamed for somehow bringing the disease down on themselves through some emotional or psychological personality trait.

In a recent study of several hundred women given the same treatments at the same stage of disease, my colleagues and I found no correlation between levels of psychological distress at the beginning of treatment and survival rates 15 years later (see Figure 12.1). Three other extensive studies—of parents who had lost a child, of spouses who had lost a mate and of people suffering chronic depression—similarly found no increase in cancer mortality over a 10-year span.

On the other hand, depression and other mood disorders obviously diminish quality of life. Numerous studies have shown that cancer can be made more bearable by psychological interventions, irrespective of the particular theoretical approaches or whether they involved group therapy or individual

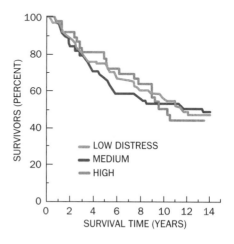

**Figure 12.1 DISTRESS LEVELS of women treated for early breast cancer show no significant correlation with survival rates in a study by Jimmie C. Holland and others.**

# Guidelines for Coping with Cancer

1.  Do not believe the old adage "cancer equals death." Today many cancers are curable; others can be controlled for long periods, during which new treatments may become available.

2.  Do not believe that you caused your cancer. There is no evidence linking specific personalities, emotional states or painful life events to the development of cancer.

3.  Do rely on strategies that helped you solve problems in the past, such as gathering information, talking to others and finding ways to feel in control. Seek help if they don't work.

4.  Do not feel guilty if you can't keep a "positive" attitude all the time. Low periods will occur, no matter how good you are at coping. There is no evidence that those periods have a negative effect on your health. If they become too frequent or severe, though, seek help.

5.  Do use support and self-help groups if they make you feel better. Leave any that make you feel worse.

6.  Do not be embarrassed to seek counsel from a mental health professional. It is a sign of strength, not weakness, and it may help you to tolerate your symptoms and treatments better.

7.  Do use any methods that aid you in gaining control over your emotions, such as meditation and relaxation.

8.  Do find a doctor of whom you can ask questions and with whom you feel mutual respect and trust. Insist on being a partner with him or her in your treatment. Ask what side effects you may expect and be prepared for them. Anticipating problems often makes them easier to handle when they occur.

9.  Do not keep your worries a secret from the person closest to you. Ask this person to accompany you to visits to the doctor when treatments are to be discussed. Research shows that you often don't hear or absorb information when you are very anxious; a second person will help you to interpret what was said.

10. Do reexplore spiritual and religious beliefs and practices that may have helped you in the past. They may comfort you and even help you find meaning in the experience of illness.

11. Do not abandon your treatment in favor of an alternative method. Discuss the benefits and risks of any alternative treatments brought to your attention with someone you trust who can assess them more objectively.

sessions. A meta-analysis of 45 controlled studies of a range of psychosocial interventions showed a positive effect on psychological well-being, though not on survival.

Yet several investigations have shown lower mortality in individuals with supportive social relationships, as compared with those lacking such ties (see Figure 12.2). Two small controlled studies done in 1989 and 1993, one of patients with

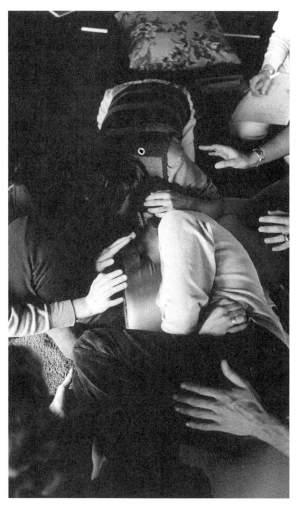

**Figure 12.2 SUPPORTIVE RELATIONSHIPS, whether involving families, religious organizations or support groups (such as the one pictured here practicing touch therapy) can improve quality of life. According to tentative findings, social support may even extend life for some cancer patients.**

melanoma (observed just after surgical removal) and one of women with advanced breast cancer, showed a positive effect not only on quality of life but also on length of survival.

Researchers are now trying to replicate these intriguing findings in larger, more tightly controlled studies. In the meantime, investigators have focused on how supportive relationships might improve patients' health. One possibility is that comforting relationships influence the immune or endocrine systems. Another hypothesis is that family members, friends and others may help patients adhere to treatment, switch to a healthier diet and take other steps that prolong life.

## Sources of Support

The family is usually the most important source of psychological support for a cancer patient. Having a physician who is knowledgeable, accessible and compassionate is also invaluable. Friends and organizations in the community provide the next level of support, and religious groups and clergy can offer solace as well. Self-help groups and professionally led groups for cancer patients, now common in most communities, help individuals to feel less alone, to share feelings with others who understand and to observe how different people cope with the same problems. Members can also exchange information about treatment, hospitals and other aspects of their care.

Group therapy is not for everyone. Some people are reluctant to share private feelings or are upset by hearing the problems of others. They may choose individual psychotherapy to deal with illness-related crises. Others may prefer approaches such as relaxation exercises, including meditation, hypnosis or yoga. Learning these techniques can alleviate anxiety, insomnia and pain by reducing muscle tension and promoting a calm, contemplative emotional state.

In advanced stages of cancer, both physical symptoms and psychological distress increase, and the emphasis of caregivers should shift from curative treatments to comfort. Patients may receive this so-called palliative care in hospitals, hospices or at home. At these stages of illness, the patient—and his or her loved ones—is in even greater need of psychological support.

Hard as it may be to believe, not all survivors of cancer view their experience in a negative light.

## The Worried Well

One growing population facing cancer-related psychological challenges are the "worried well," who recognize that their genetic history indicates an increased risk of cancer. Our studies of women at risk for breast cancer found that many were so anxious that they did not take the proper steps for diagnosing the disease early, such as getting regular mammograms (see figure at right). Others have taken drastic steps, such as having prophylactic mastectomies that were not consonant with their actual risk. The recent development of genetic tests for cancer raises questions about when such tests should be given, how the results should be conveyed to a carrier of a cancer-linked gene and how that person should be counseled thereafter. Public health policies must be carefully crafted to ensure that patients are aided rather than harmed by this emerging technology.

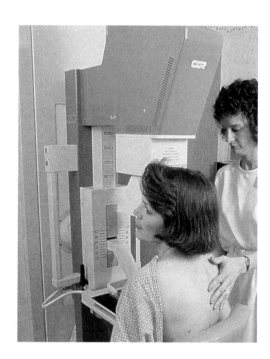

Some have told me, "I know it sounds crazy, but I'm glad I had cancer. The experience changed my life for the better." Confrontation with serious illness leads some people to grow emotionally and thus to attempt to correct long-standing problems or to explore areas of life that they had never had time for previously. For the many others who cannot be so sanguine about their experience, there may still be ways to reduce its devastating psychological impact. The days in which cancer patients had to suffer alone and in silence are over.

# Alternative Cancer Treatments

*Miraculous cures are a myth, but some regimens may well improve the quality of life for patients.*

. . .

Jean-Jacques Aulas

C onventional therapy for cancer is generally painful and debilitating. Far too often, it is also ineffective or prolongs survival for only a short time. It is not surprising, therefore, that people faced with the prospect of suffering and death are drawn to alternative therapies touted to be more gentle or more effective, or both. Yet whether to choose alternative therapies poses the sharpest of dilemmas for patients, because the unconventional options generally have not been proved effective by standard evaluative procedures and may turn out to be costly, useless or even dangerous—shortening lives rather than extending them.

It is hard to say exactly how many cancer patients turn to alternative medicine. Surveys have come up with numbers between about 15 and 25 percent. Such figures are undoubtedly underestimated; at least 30 percent of patients contacted in the surveys declined interviews. Interestingly, about three quarters of those seeking alternative medicine said they had not informed their physicians, and the vast majority continued to undergo conventional treatment. Malcolm L. Brigden of Metro-McNair Clinical Laboratories in British

Columbia has estimated that roughly half of all cancer patients seek such therapy.

French physician Olivier Jallut has documented more than 80 unconventional medical techniques, ranging from acupressure to macrobiotic Zen. These methods can be divided into two major groups: those used for diagnosis and those intended to treat cancers.

None of the alternative diagnostic tools has a rational basis. Many consist of a mixed bag of general laboratory tests and sorcery, and not one has shown the least official value for detecting any form of cancer. I believe these techniques should be banned or that the "institutes" that use them should supply prospective patients with objective information about their effectiveness.

The status of alternative therapies is less clear-cut. Few have been tested in controlled clinical trials—currently the only way of documenting the efficacy and safety of a particular treatment. Laetrile and high-dose vitamin C are among the few that have been tested in this way; neither was found to be more effective than a placebo. Other therapies, such as "antineoplastons" (peptide molecules isolated by the independent cancer researcher Stanislaw R.

# A Look at Some Alternative Treatments

ANTINEOPLASTONS are peptides (bits of protein) that their discoverer, Stanislaw R. Burzynski of the Burzynski Research Institute in Houston, asserts can slow or reverse tumor growth. The National Cancer Institute (NCI) started a clinical trial of antineoplaston therapy in 1993; the project foundered when Burzynski and NCI investigators disagreed on treatment protocols and criteria for selecting patients.

GERSON THERAPY, after Max B. Gerson, is based on hourly consumption of crushed fruits and vegetables to correct alleged physiological imbalances. Coffee enemas are given to remove dead cells and toxins, and patients receive nutritional supplements as well. Several independent evaluations of case records have concluded that it has no discernible effectiveness.

HYDRAZINE SULFATE, a compound studied in Leningrad for more than 20 years, may reverse cachexia, the wasting of cancer patients' bodies. Modest improvements in survival (but no remissions) have been documented.

ORTHOMOLECULAR THERAPY, originally developed by the late Nobelist Linus Pauling, requires consumption of megadoses of vitamin C in an effort to aid the body's repair systems. NCI-sponsored trials did not demonstrate any superiority to placebos.

PSYCHOLOGICAL INTERVENTIONS (including Simonton therapy, after O. Carl Simonton, and Bernard S. Siegel's Exceptional Cancer Patients program) use combinations of meditation, visualization, therapy, support groups and other exercises. No definitive studies of their impact on survival have been conducted. Some physicians accept these techniques as adjuncts to conventional cancer therapy because they enhance patients' sense of well-being.

**714X** is a proprietary injection said to contain compounds that mobilize the immune system against cancer. Samples analyzed by the Food and Drug Administration contained only camphor and water.

Sources: *Unconventional Cancer Treatments* (OTA Report No. OTA-H-405, 1990), Boston University Medical Center alternative cancer treatment Web site: http://web.bu.edu/COHIS/cancer/about/alttx/about.htm

Burzynski, who asserts that they have a powerful antitumor effect), have been slated for testing, but trials have foundered as conventional and unconventional researchers argue over the proper guidelines for enrolling and treating patients. In short, no alternative treatment has been clearly shown to induce tumor regression or to increase survival.

Many doctors and patients have made claims for so-called complementary therapies—that is, nutritional and psychological treatments that patients undergo in conjunction with conventional treatments. Even if a cancer is not cured, they assert, patients' quality of life may be improved and survival prolonged. It is difficult to conduct randomized trials of psychological interventions or large-scale changes in life patterns, so there are as yet no definitive data that demonstrate advantages in either quality of life or survival. Some preliminary studies have reported that breast cancer patients receiving psychotherapy or enrolled in support groups survived roughly a year longer than those who had no such aids; quality of life

# How to Evaluate Alternative Therapies for Cancer

Ideally, prospective patients would be able to tell whether an alternative cancer treatment was likely to help them by looking at the results of randomized clinical trials carried out on people with their particular malignancy. But most unconventional therapies have not been studied in such careful detail.

In 1992 the National Cancer Institute set up a program to evaluate alternative medicines. Its guidelines for patients are heavily weighted toward conventional oncology, but they offer a useful starting point. If the answer is "yes" to any but the first of the following questions, the NCI says, prospective patients should be on their guard:

- Has the treatment been evaluated in clinical trials?
- Do the practitioners of an approach claim that the medical community is trying to keep their cure from the public?
- Does the treatment rely on nutritional or diet therapy as its main focus?
- Do those who endorse the treatment claim that it is harmless and painless and that it produces no unpleasant side effects?
- Does the treatment have a "secret formula" that only a small group of practitioners can use?

Another important step in assessing the possible value of unconventional therapy is making sure that cancer is present in the first place. Doctors reviewing the medical records of patients ostensibly cured by alternative treatments have in some cases been unable to find any solid evidence (such as examination of cells removed in a biopsy) that malignancies had ever existed.

If abnormal cells are present, it is crucial to determine their potential for malignancy and the likely prognosis. Patients whose cancers are treatable by surgery, radiation or chemotherapy should not pursue alternative treatments first.

Many patients undertake alternative courses of treatment in conjunction with mainstream medical care, so it appears that the other options may answer a different need than those addressed by traditional oncology. Studies of some psychological interventions (ranging from support groups to psychotherapy to "visualization") have suggested that patients may experience better quality of life even if their survival time is not definitively increased. Only patients and their families can decide precisely what they want from a particular course of treatment—conventional or alternative.

was also apparently enhanced. Similar, potentially encouraging results have come from early investigations of dietary regimens that concentrate on reducing or eliminating meat intake and consuming large quantities of fresh vegetables in an attempt to bolster the body's response to cancer.

Mainstream epidemiologic studies have demonstrated correlations between proper nutrition and mortality as well as between social and psychological well-being and health. It would therefore not be surprising if such factors should affect the survival of cancer patients. Yet not all therapies are benign. For example, some macrobiotic diets are deficient enough in nutrients that they have clearly visible adverse effects on frail patients.

## Making Decisions

Although no alternative treatment for cancer has a definite influence on the course of the disease, there are nonetheless situations in which complementary methods may be helpful. Indeed, many physicians recommend psychosocial and nutritional interventions. I see no reason to avoid such options, including acupuncture, homeopathy and trace-element supplementation.

If conventional treatments have been exhausted, unconventional ones may increase patients' sense of control and well-being even if they do not lengthen survival. Furthermore, even during the course of a serious disease the placebo effect—essentially a patient's belief in the efficacy of treatment—can relieve pain, anxiety and other functional disorders that accompany cancer. As a result, some patients attracted to these treatments may benefit in some way.

The chosen method must be absolutely safe, however, and it must not replace conventional treatments that have documented efficacy. Cancer is a highly variable disease, and some forms are in fact curable. It would be a tragedy if patients with juvenile leukemia or Hodgkin's lymphoma died because they had picked an alternative medication over a well-tested conventional therapy.

# Controlling the Pain of Cancer

*Despite enormous advances in treating pain, many cancer patients still suffer needlessly. Some simple practices can make a difference.*

• • •

Kathleen M. Foley

Pain is one of the most feared consequences of cancer—and with good reason. Studies in the United States have shown that at least one third of all cancer patients undergoing chemotherapy or other antitumor treatments and two thirds of those with advanced cancer suffer significant discomfort. Providing relief is vital not only as an end in itself but also to improve the patient's prospects for survival. Pain can erode a patient's willingness to continue treatment, even to live.

Decades of research and clinical experience have yielded a wide variety of methods for diagnosing and managing the various types of cancer-related pain. Drugs can now be delivered not just orally and intravenously but also through suppositories, skin patches, bedside pumps, implanted pumps and topical creams. Researchers have reached a better understanding of why tumors that have invaded bones or the nervous system generate so much pain, and they have tailored treatments to each process.

Physicians have improved their ability to measure levels of painkilling medications in body fluids and to correlate these levels with patients' reported sense of relief. They have also devised drug-delivery protocols designed to stop pain before it starts. All these advances serve to maximize relief while minimizing drug side effects, such as grogginess, constipation and nausea.

Moreover, investigators have come to understand how a person's state of mind—and perception of his or her own condition—can affect the experience of pain. For example, those who have undergone surgery with a high likelihood of eliminating the disease may regard their acute but transitory pain as more bearable than do patients with chronic pain from more advanced disease. Depression can also exacerbate perception of pain. Prescribing antidepressants can thus alleviate both psychological and physical discomfort.

Clinicians have found innovative ways to help patients describe accurately the ebb and flow of both physical pain and psychological distress. For example, very young children and others who have trouble communicating verbally can indicate their level of distress by pointing to one in a series of cartoon faces whose expressions range from no pain to agonizing pain.

Although some types of pain resist treatment, studies indicate that as many as 95 percent of cancer

# Getting Doctors to Listen

Recently a group at the Dartmouth-Hitchcock Medical Center created an interactive video-disk to teach medical professionals how to provide pain relief—and to motivate them to do so. The disk, not yet available, makes its case in part with a moving testimonial by Claudia Graves, a 42-year-old woman with recurrent breast cancer.

Graves said the pain caused by both her cancer and her treatments gradually worsened during the course of the illness, affecting her relationships with her friends and four children. Her doctors, while aware that she was in pain, seemed not to understand how it was affecting her. One day when she went to the hospital for radiation treatment "there was another doctor I hadn't seen before, and I was really able to explain the pain to him."

The physician arranged an appointment with a neurologist, who suggested that Graves try morphine. She had feared that she would become addicted or seem "drugged" or that she would lose her ability to think clearly. But the drug eased her pain without these side effects.

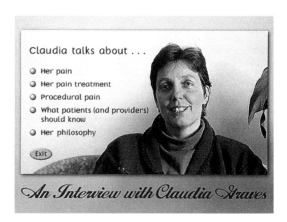

Claudia talks about . . .
- Her pain
- Her pain treatment
- Procedural pain
- What patients (and providers) should know
- Her philosophy

Exit

*An Interview with Claudia Graves*

"I'm not foggy-headed. I can think and enjoy my children and my relationships with friends."

The most important lesson she learned is that patients or family members must "really insist that the medical team stop and listen," Graves said. "Any cancer patient deserves a doctor who will listen, who treats the patient as part of the team."

---

patients can get relief if properly medicated. Tragically, many continue to suffer needlessly. A 1994 study found that 42 percent of a group of cancer patients received inadequate pain treatment. The elderly, less educated and those with lower incomes were most likely to have been undermedicated. A 1993 survey of 1,177 American physicians found that 85 percent, who had cared for more than 70,000 people with cancer during the previous six months, provided inadequate relief for the majority of those in pain.

What accounts for the astonishing gap between the degree of relief that is possible and the suffering that still persists in reality? Sadly, the effort to improve the management of pain has been enormously complicated by the so-called war on drugs. The years of antidrug campaigns have left both the public and health care professionals with greatly exaggerated fears about the risks of opioids, which are still the most effective known painkillers.

Many studies have shown that the medical use of analgesic drugs is safe and does not cause psychological addiction in those who had not previously shown such tendencies. Even when patients can administer the drug themselves with bedside pumps, they rarely deliver more than they need to suppress their pain. Those who receive such drugs may become physically dependent—that is, the drug must be withdrawn slowly to prevent symptoms of withdrawal. This state is very different, however, from true addiction, which is characterized by constant craving and compulsive drug-seeking behavior.

Poor communication between physicians and patients is another major obstacle to assessment and treatment of pain. Too often physicians attribute a complaint about pain to psychological factors. Patients' attitudes compound the problem. Like physicians, many patients have exaggerated fears of the risks of painkillers, and they often believe that "good" patients should not complain.

# Painkillers for Cancer

| DRUGS | BENEFITS | SIDE EFFECTS* |
|---|---|---|
| **Nonopiods**<br>Acetaminophen, aspirin, ibuprofen | Can control mild to moderate pain; some versions can be bought without prescription | Can cause slow blood clotting and upset stomach, bleeding in the stomach and kidney problems |
| **Opioids**<br>Morphine, hydromorphone, oxycodone, codeine, fentanyl, methadones | Can control moderate to severe pain without bleeding | Can cause constipation, sleepiness, nausea and vomiting, itchiness and urinary problems; may also slow breathing when first taken |
| **Antidepressants**<br>Amitriptyline, imipramine | Can help control tingling or burning pain from nerve injury; may improve sleep | Can cause dry mouth, sleepiness, constipation and dizziness on standing up suddenly |
| **Anticonvulsants**<br>Carbamazepine, phenytoin | Can help control tingling or burning from nerve injury | Can affect liver and blood cell function |
| **Steroids**<br>Prednisone, dexamethasone | Can help relieve bone pain and pain caused by spinal cord and brain tumors | May cause confusion, fluid buildup, bleeding and irritation in stomach |

* Usually can be minimized
Source: National Cancer Institute

Recent studies of medical students, physicians, nurses and state medical boards have also demonstrated a significant lack of theoretical and practical knowledge about analgesic drug therapy for cancer pain. These deficiencies reflect not caregivers' lack of compassion but rather flaws in the health care education and delivery systems. Obviously, knowledge about managing pain needs to be better integrated into medical education at all levels.

But communication and education are not enough. Hospitals and other medical institutions must integrate pain management into routine practice. One step is to make physicians and nurses accountable for relieving patients' pain. The threat of legal sanctions may provide extra motivation; ethicists have argued that excessive pain, resulting from substandard treatment, constitutes medical negligence. Patients and family members must also learn how to talk to doctors about pain and to insist on treatment. Reading the publications listed at the end of this section under "Finding More Information" may help.

Research has shown that having even one recognized pain expert serving as a role model in a hospital or other institution can help transform knowledge into practice. Another important step, advocated by the American Pain Society, is called "making pain visible." This approach calls for recording pain intensity on a patient's vital-sign sheet as a routine practice. Pain is much more likely to be treated if it is consistently measured and recorded.

Fortunately, the need for better pain control is beginning to be recognized in the United States and internationally. The American Pain Society, the American Society of Clinical Oncology and the Oncology Nursing Society have all issued guidelines for the treatment of cancer pain, as well as pain management curricula for medical schools. Almost every state has an initiative to increase awareness about cancer pain among both caregivers and the public. At the federal level, the National Cancer Institute, the American Cancer Society and the Agency for Health Care Policy and Research have all supported efforts to improve pain treatment for cancer. The World Health Organization has created the Cancer Pain Relief Program, the goal of which is summarized by the slogan "Freedom from Cancer Pain." It is an attainable—and morally imperative—goal.

# Current Controversy:
# What Are Obstacles to Ideal Care?

W. Wayt Gibbs

Shari R. Kahane was suckling her second child when she first felt an ominous twinge in her breast. Her gynecologist ascribed the abnormal pain to a nursing infection, a common cause. Kahane, a 43-year-old emergency room physician in Calabasas, Calif., was skeptical. But when she saw two other doctors, they agreed; in their palpations and mammograms, neither physician detected anything unusual. "So I believed what they told me," Kahane says.

Her trust was dangerously misplaced, for all three doctors missed a cancer that had taken root in her chest and was spreading. Misdiagnoses were only the start of her ordeal; in Kahane's subsequent struggle to get a lifesaving experimental treatment, she also had to overcome the ignorance of some charged with her care and the bureaucracy and costs of cutting-edge medicine. These obstacles, many oncologists and patient advocates report, often stymie those who are less educated, persistent and lucky than Kahane. As a result, the quality of cancer care can vary dramatically from patient to patient.

Kahane's pain subsided, but nagging doubts returned. One night, after seeing a knowledgeable gynecologist on a PBS television special, Kahane decided to track her down. "She agreed to examine me—and she found a cyst," Kahane recalls. Although a biopsy taken through a needle found no malignancy, Kahane's radiologist insisted the lump be removed anyway. During her surgery, the hospital lab issued a clear report: no cancer. Relieved, Kahane went home, only to learn days later that the lab had made a mistake. She sought a second surgeon, who reopened her chest and discovered cancer not only in her breast but also in 11 lymph nodes.

"We don't really know how often misdiagnosis occurs, but doctors and cancer patients are very concerned," states Allen S. Lichter, who chairs the public issues committee for the American Society of Clinical Oncology (ASCO). Part of the worry, he says, focuses on health maintenance organizations (HMOs), where physicians can refuse to refer patients to specialists. "We are pushing the idea of report cards on HMOs' cancer care that will measure the average stage [of disease] at diagnosis and the delay before seeing a specialist."

Of course, specialists are only as helpful as they are knowledgeable. Cancer treatments evolve quickly; some physicians fall behind. Kahane says her first surgeon—chief of surgery at a large Los

Angeles hospital—told her she had no chance of survival: standard chemotherapy would buy her only a few more months. Although Kahane knew such bleak prognoses are often correct, she remained unconvinced. Digging through journals, she found reports on a relatively new treatment, combining high-dose chemotherapy with stem cell transplants, that in one trial had more than doubled the number of patients surviving for three years. Not until Kahane reached her fourth specialist did she find someone who knew about the therapy and would help her get into a trial.

Many patients do not even know that being in a clinical trial is an option, which is one reason why only 2 to 3 percent of cancer patients in the United States participate in clinical studies. "It takes us several years to fill a study, when it should take half or a third of that time," Lichter says. "If we could get 10 percent of cancer patients involved, we could answer more questions and answer them much faster."

But many oncologists complain that insurance companies, especially managed care plans such as HMOs, are trying to cut costs by refusing to reimburse for unproved therapies, clinical trials and even new drugs. In a 1993 survey 856 oncologists reported that more than 3,300 of their patients were kept out of trials because their insurers refused to pay. That is a shame, Lichter says, because although experimental treatments involve unknown risks, "data suggest that patients who participate in clinical trials can have better—sometimes significantly better—outcomes than those who get standard therapy."

Patients may never know what they are missing. "HMOs in most states can have gag rules that prohibit physicians from telling patients about any treatment options that are not covered," Kahane points out.

"It is shortsighted to deny benefits [for experimental therapies]," argues Joseph S. Bailes, who chairs the ASCO's clinical practice committee. "Most advances in oncology come in the form of new drugs, so progress depends on clinical trials." Even more worrisome, he says, is that an increasing number—already more than a third—of insurance plans are refusing to add newly approved cancer drugs to the list of those they cover.

Since March 1996, when the Food and Drug Administration announced that it was lowering its efficacy standards for cancer drugs and clearing the backlog of those awaiting approval, several new agents have made it to market. Yet more than half the medicines used to treat cancer are prescribed "off-label"—that is, to treat a condition for which they have not been approved. The growth factors Kahane needed to support her regenerating bone marrow, for example, were then unapproved for breast cancer. Now they are used off-label to treat ovarian cancer.

Medicare, which covers more than half of all cancer patients, began covering most off-label prescriptions in 1994, but Bailes says fewer than 12 states have laws requiring private insurers to do the same. Several bills now before Congress would rectify that and would allow drug companies to distribute peer-reviewed studies of unapproved uses for their products.

Thanks to Kahane's skepticism, perseverance and good fortune, she is healthy—30 months after her diagnosis. "I recently ran into that chief surgeon at the gym," she recounts. "When he saw me running four miles on the treadmill, his teeth nearly hit the floor. You know, he still didn't know about stem cell therapy. If I'd listened to him, I'd probably be dead now," she says, before dashing off to pick up her children.

# Finding More Information

• • •

W. Wayt Gibbs

Fortunately, access to incisive knowledge about cancer and its treatment is easier to obtain than ever before. The catch is knowing what information can be trusted. This problem is particularly acute on the Internet, where only a fraction of what is on-line is true, accurate, reliable and up-to-date.

The following resources serve as a good starting point for beginning a search for more information. When using the World Wide Web, remember that interlinked sites are not always equally trustworthy. Patients should discuss the information they find with their health care providers.

—The Editors of SCIENTIFIC AMERICAN

## Resources Available by Telephone and On-line

**American Cancer Society**
1599 Clifton Road NE, Atlanta, GA 30329
*by phone:* 800-227-2345. Outside the U.S.,
call 404-320-3333
*via the Web:* http://www.cancer.org/
The Web site has abundant and authoritative information about the treatment, prevention and detection of cancer. Patients and their families can also learn about a range of other services available to them, including financial assistance, household help, job rehabilitation, dietary advice and hospice services.

**CancerGuide: Steve Dunn's Cancer Information Page**
*via the Web:* http://www.cancerguide.org/
Dunn, a cancer survivor, maintains this remarkably helpful page, which offers links to other good resources, as well as advice about how to make the best use of that information.

**Cancer Information Service**
National Cancer Institute (NCI)
Office of Cancer Communications
31 Center Drive, Building 31, Room 10A07,
Bethesda, MD 20892
*by phone:* 800-4-CANCER (800-422-6237)
This phone service provides extensive information on treatment options, screening, prevention, supportive care, clinical trials, newly approved anticancer drugs and many drugs under investigation, as well as directories of physicians and care organizations. It draws on excellent resources, including the computerized Physician Data Query (PDQ) database compiled by the NCI's International Cancer Information Center. The content of the PDQ is peer-reviewed regularly by boards of cancer experts and is updated monthly.

**CancerNet/CancerLit**
National Cancer Institute
*by fax-on-demand:* 301-402-5874 (call first using the

handset of your fax machine, then follow the instructions)

*by e-mail:* cancernet@icicc.nci.nih.gov (place the word "help" in the body of the message for a reply containing a table of contents and further instructions)

*via the Web:* CancerNet—http://wwwicic.nci.nih.gov/ CancerLit—http: //wwwicic.nci.nih.gov/canlit/canlit.htm

The data in CancerNet, which includes the PDQ database, are conveniently sorted for access by the general public, health care providers and researchers, so users may choose the level most appropriate for them. The page for CancerLit, the NCI's bibliographic database of published research, has compilations of select citations and abstracts on various cancer topics.

## CANSearch: A Guide to Cancer Resources on the Internet

National Coalition for Cancer Survivorship
1010 Wayne Avenue, Suite 505, Silver Spring, MD 20910
*by phone:* 301-650-8868
*by fax:* 301-565-9670
*via the Web:* http: //www.access.digex.net/~mkragen/cansearch.html

The CANSearch site helps to guide patients and their families to reliable sources of information on-line.

## The National Alliance of Breast Cancer Organizations (NABCO)

9 East 37th Street, 10th Floor, New York, NY 10016
*by phone:* 800-719-9154
*via the Web:* http://www.nabco.org/

NABCO is a coalition of more than 370 organizations across the U.S. that offer detection services, treatment and care to breast cancer patients. It also provides information about clinical trials and breast cancer support groups.

## OncoLink: The University of Pennsylvania Cancer Center Resource

*via the Web:* http://cancer.med.upenn.edu/

This well-organized, comprehensive site can be of use to both patients and medical professionals seeking information.

## The Prostate Cancer InfoLink

*via the Web:*

http://www.comed.com/prostate/

This resource is a good place to turn for information about prostate cancer screening, diagnosis, treatment and support.

## The Skin Cancer Foundation

P.O. Box 561, New York, NY 10156
*by phone:* 800-SKIN-490 (800-754-6490)

The Foundation offers numerous brochures, books and newsletters on skin cancer.

## TeleSCAN: Telematics Services in Cancer

*via the Web:* http://telescan.nki.nl/

This Europe-based site offers a variety of information services to the general public, physicians and researchers, including bulletin boards where patients can converse and lists of clinical trials in Europe.

## Books and Periodicals

Although textbooks and technical journals are aimed at physicians and researchers rather than general readers, some patients still like to consult these sources. The following items can be found in many medical, university or hospital libraries. Keep in mind that journals often present results from early trials; these findings cannot be applied readily or reliably to patients in general.

**Periodicals:**
*Cancer* (American Cancer Society). John Wiley & Sons.
*The Cancer Journal* from Scientific American.
*The Journal of Clinical Oncology: Official Journal of the American Society of Clinical Oncology.* W. B. Saunders.
*Oncology Times: The Independent Newspaper for Cancer Specialists.* Lippincott-Raven.

**Textbooks:**
*American Cancer Society Textbook of Clinical Oncology,* 2nd edition. American Cancer Society, 1995.
*Cancer: Principles and Practice of Oncology,* 5th edition. Edited by Vincent T. DeVita, Jr., Samuel Hellman and Steven A. Rosenberg. J. B. Lippincott, 1996.
*Clinical Oncology.* Edited by Martin A. Abeloff, James O. Armitage, Allen S. Lichter and John E. Niederhuber. Churchill Livingstone, 1995.

# The Authors

...

**JOHN RENNIE** and **RICKI RUSTING** ("Introduction: Making Headway Against Cancer") are editor in chief and associate editor, respectively, of SCIENTIFIC AMERICAN.

**ROBERT A. WEINBERG** ("How Cancer Arises") is Member of the Whitehead Institute for Biomedical Research and a professor of biology at the Massachusetts Institute of Technology, where he earned his doctoral degree in biology in 1969. His laboratory was instrumental in isolating the first human oncogene and the first human tumor suppressor gene. Weinberg, a member of the National Academy of Sciences, has won many awards for his contributions to the understanding of cancer genetics, most recently the G. H. A. Clowes Memorial Award of the American Association for Cancer Research.

**ERKKI RUOSLAHTI** ("How Cancer Spreads") is president and chief executive officer of the Burnham Institute (formerly the La Jolla Cancer Research Foundation) in La Jolla, Calif., and adjunct professor in pathology at the University of California, San Diego. Born in Finland, he attended the University of Helsinki, where he received his bachelor's degree in 1961, his medical degree in 1965 and his medical doctorate in immunology in 1967. He has been the recipient of many internationally respected honors; in 1995 he was a Nobel Fellow at the Karolinska Institute and delivered a Nobel Forum Lecture.

**DIMITRIOS TRICHOPOULOS, FREDERICK P. LI** and **DAVID J. HUNTER** ("What Causes Cancer?") are colleagues at Harvard University. Trichopoulos is director of the Harvard Center for Cancer Prevention at the School of Public Health, professor of epidemiology and the Vincent L. Gregory Professor of Cancer Prevention. He was born in Athens, Greece. Li, who was born in China, is professor of medicine at Harvard Medical School and professor of clinical cancer epidemiology at the School of Public Health. Hunter, a native of Australia, is associate professor of epidemiology at the School of Public Health and executive director of the Center for Cancer Prevention.

**LORI MILLER KASE** (the box "Why Community Cancer Clusters Are Often Ignored") is a science and health writer based in Virginia.

**WALTER C. WILLETT, GRAHAM A. COLDITZ** and **NANCY E. MUELLER** ("Strategies for Minimizing Cancer Risk") are colleagues at Harvard University. Willett is chairman of the department of nutrition and professor of epidemiology in the School of Public Health, professor in the Medical School and associate physician at Brigham and Women's Hospital in Boston. Colditz is associate professor in the Medical School and associate director for education at the Harvard Center for Cancer Prevention. Mueller is professor of epidemiology in the School of Public Health and a member of the board of scientific advisers for the National Cancer Institute.

**PETER GREENWALD** ("Chemoprevention of Cancer") has been director of the National Cancer Institute's division of cancer prevention and control since its inception in 1981. Previously, he directed the cancer control bureau and then the division of epidemiology in the New York State Department of Health. He has held appointments at Albany Medical College, Rensselaer Polytechnic Institute and Memorial Sloan-Kettering Institute for Cancer Research.

**KAREN WRIGHT** (the box "A Plea for Prevention") is a science and health writer based in New Hampshire.

**NANCY E. DAVIDSON** ("Current Controversy: Is Hormone Replacement Therapy a Risk?") holds the Breast Cancer Research chair in Oncology at the Johns Hopkins Oncology Center.

**DAVID SIDRANSKY** ("Advances in Cancer Detection") holds joint appointments at Johns Hopkins University School of Medicine as associate professor of oncology and of otolaryngology (with a specialty in head and neck surgery) and of cellular and molecular medicine. He is also director of the head and neck cancer research division there. He serves as editor of the journals *Predictive Oncology, Clinical Cancer Research* and *Cancer Research.* Sidransky has a research agreement with Oncor. He received his medical degree from the Baylor College of Medicine in Houston in 1984.

**GARY STIX** (the box "Is Genetic Testing Premature?") is a staff writer at SCIENTIFIC AMERICAN.

**MARYELLEN L. GIGER** and **CHARLES A. PELIZZARI** ("Advances in Tumor Imaging") pursue complementary lines of research at the University of Chicago School of Medicine. Giger is an associate professor in the department of radiology; she received her Ph.D. in medical physics from the University of Chicago in 1985. Pelizzati is an associate professor in the department of radiation and cellular oncology; he received his Ph.D. in nuclear engineering from the University of Michigan in 1974.

**GINA MARANTO** ("Current Controversy: Should Women in Their 40s Have Mammograms?") is a science and health writer based in Florida.

**GERALD E. HANKS** and **PETER T. SCARDINO** ("Current Controversy: Does Screening for Prostate Cancer Make Sense?") specialize in prostate cancer research. Hanks is chair of the department of radiation oncology at the Fox

Chase Cancer Center in Philadelphia. Scardino is chair of the department of urology at the Baylor College of Medicine in Houston.

**SAMUEL HELLMAN** and **EVERETT E. VOKES** ("Advancing Current Treatments for Cancer") are professors at the University of Chicago. Before joining the department of radiation and cellular oncology at Chicago in 1988, Hellman worked in New York City as a professor and physician in chief at Memorial Sloan-Kettering Cancer Center and as a professor of radiation oncology at Cornell University Medical College. Vokes received training at the University of Bonn Medical School in West Germany. He completed internships at Bonn and Chicago, as well as a residency at the University of Southern California Los Angeles County Hospital, before undertaking a fellowship in hematology and oncology at Chicago in 1983. Four years later he became a professor there in the department of medicine and now serves the university's cancer center as associate director for clinical affairs. Hellman and Vokes both have published and lectured widely about their research on cancer therapy.

**KAREN ANTMAN** ("Current Controversy: When Are Bone Marrow Transplants Considered?") is director of the Columbia-Presbyterian Comprehensive Cancer Center at Columbia University.

**LLOYD J. OLD** ("Immunotherapy for Cancer") received his medical degree in 1958 from the University of California, San Francisco. He then joined the Memorial Sloan-Kettering Institute for Cancer Research, where he became associate director of research from 1973 to 1983. Old is now director and CEO of the Ludwig Institute for Cancer Research in New York City.

**ALLEN OLIFF, JACKSON B. GIBBS** and **FRANK McCORMICK** ("New Molecular Targets for Cancer Therapy") are pharmaceutical researchers seeking remedies for cancer on the molecular level. Oliff, who received his M.D. from the Albert Einstein College of Medicine in the Bronx, N.Y., is executive director for cancer research at Merck Research Laboratories in West Point, Pa. He has served on several academic and professional advisory boards, including that of the National Cancer Institute. Gibbs is Merck's senior director of cancer research and holds an adjunct professorship at the University of Pennsylvania School of Medicine. He received his Ph.D. from the University of Virginia and serves on various editorial and advisory boards. McCormick founded Onyx Pharmaceuticals in Richmond, Calif., in 1992 and serves as its chief scientific officer. He earned his Ph.D. from the University of Cambridge and worked as vice president for research at Cetus Corporation and Chiron Corporation.

**JUDAH FOLKMAN** ("Fighting Cancer by Attacking Its Blood Supply") is director of the surgical research laboratory at Children's Hospital Medical Center of Harvard Medical School. His laboratory reported the first purified angiogenic molecule and the first angiogenesis inhibitor. Folkman's group then proposed the concept of angiogenic disease. Folkman is a fellow of the American Academy of Arts and Sciences and a member of the National Academy of Sciences.

**JIMMIE C. HOLLAND** ("Cancer's Psychological Challenges") is chief of the psychiatry service and Wayne E. Chapman Chair of Psychiatric Oncology at the Memorial Sloan-Kettering Cancer Center in New York City. She is also professor of psychiatry and vice chair of the department of psychiatry at Cornell University Medical College.

**JEAN-JACQUES AULAS** ("Alternative Cancer Treatments") has studied the claims of alternative medicine for more than 10 years. He is a psychiatrist and pharmacologist at the Clinical Unit of Biological Psychiatry in CHS "Le Vinatier" de Lyon-Bron and associate editor of *Revue Prescrire,* an independent French monthly medical publication.

**KATHLEEN M. FOLEY** ("Controlling the Pain of Cancer") has dedicated her career to treating pain. She is chief of the Pain Service in the department of neurology at Memorial Sloan-Kettering Cancer Center in New York City as well as professor of neurology, neuroscience and clinical pharmacology at the Cornell University Medical College. Foley is director of the Open Society Institute's Project on Death in America and of the World Health Organization's Collaborating Center for Cancer Pain Research and Education.

**W. WAYT GIBBS** ("Current Controversy: What Are Obstacles to Ideal Care?") is a staff writer at Scientific American.

# Bibliography

...

## 1. How Cancer Arises

Bishop, J. M. 1993. Cancer: The rise of the genetic paradigm. *Genes and Development* 9 (June): 1309–1315.

Cairns, J. 1978. *Cancer: Science and society.* New York: W. H. Freeman.

Cooper, G. M. 1995. *Oncogenes*, 2nd ed. Boston: Jones and Bartlett Publishers.

Varmus, H., and R. A. Weinberg. 1993. *Genes and the biology of cancer.* New York: Scientific American Library.

Vogelstein, B., and K. W. Kinzler. 1993. The multistep nature of cancer. *Trends in Genetics* 9 (April): 138–141.

## 2. How Cancer Spreads

Akiyama, S. K., K. Olden and K. M. Yamada. 1996. Fibronectin and integrins in invasion and metastasis. *Cancer and Metastasis Reviews* 14: 173–189.

Bernstein, L. R., and L. A. Liotta. 1994. Molecular mediators of interactions with extracellular matrix components in metastasis and angiogenesis. *Current Opinion in Oncology* 6 (January): 106–113.

Lewin, David I. 1996. Evolutions: Metastasis. *Journal of NIH Research* 8 (June): 82–87.

Ruoslahti, Erkki, and John C. Reed. 1994. Anchorage dependence, integrins, and apoptosis. *Cell* 77 (May 20): 477–478.

## 3. What Causes Cancer?

Schottenfeld, D., and J. F. Fraumeni, Jr., eds. 1996. *Cancer epidemiology and prevention.* New York: Oxford University Press.

Tomatis, L., ed. 1990. *Cancer: Causes, occurrence and control.* New York: Oxford University Press.

Trichopoulos, Dimitrios, L. Lipworth, E. Petridou and H. O. Adami. In press. Epidemiology of Cancer. In *Epidemiology of cancer.* Philadelphia: Lippincott-Raven.

## 4. Strategies for Minimizing Cancer Risk

Avoidable causes of cancer. 1995. Special issue of *Environmental Health Perspectives* 103, Supplement 8 (November).

Ames, Bruce N., Lois Swirsky Gold, and Walter C. Willett. 1995. The causes and prevention of cancer. *Proceedings of the National Academy of Sciences* 92 (June 6): 5258–5265.

Cairns, John. 1985. The treatment of diseases and the war against cancer. *Scientific American* 253 (November): 51–59.

Henderson, Brian E., Ronald K. Ross and Malcolm C. Pike. 1991. Toward the primary prevention of cancer. *Science* 254 (November 22): 1131–1138.

Warner, Kenneth. 1989. Smoking and health: A 25-year experience. *American Journal of Public Health* 79 (February): 141–143.

## 5. Chemoprevention of Cancer

Boone, C. W., G. J. Kelloff and V. E. Steele. 1992. Natural history of intraepithelial neoplasia in humans with implications for cancer chemopreventive strategy. *Cancer Research* 52 (April 1): 1651–1659.

El-Bayoumy, K. 1994. Evaluation of chemopreventive agents against breast cancer and proposed strategies for future clinical intervention trials. *Carcinogenesis* 15 (November): 2395–2420.

Greenwald, P., G. Kelloff, C. Burch-Whitman and B. S. Kramer. 1995. Chemoprevention. *CA Cancer Journal for Clinicians* 45 (January): 31–49.

Kelloff, G. J., et al. 1995. Approaches to the development and marketing approval of drugs that prevent cancer. *Cancer Epidemiology, Biomarkers and Prevention* 4 (January): 1–10.

Nayfield, S. G., J. E. Karp, L. G. Ford, A. Dorr and B. S. Kramer. 1991. Potential role of tamoxifen in prevention of breast cancer. *Journal of the National Cancer Institute* 83 (October 16): 1450–1459.

## 6. Advances in Cancer Detection

Holtzman, N. A. 1994. Discovery transfer and diffusion of technologies for the detection of genetic disorders: Policy implications. *International Journal of Technology Assessment in Health Care* 10 (Fall): 562–572.

Hruban, R. H., P. van der Riet, Y. S. Erozan and D. Sidransky. 1994. Molecular biology and the early detection of carcinoma of the bladder—The case of Hubert H. Humphrey. *New England Journal of Medicine* 330 (May 5): 1276–1278.

Lerman, Caryn, and Robert T. Croyle. 1996. Emotional and behavioral responses to genetic testing for susceptibility to cancer. *Oncology* 10 (February): 191–199.

Sidransky, David. 1994. Molecular screening: How long can we afford to wait? *Journal of the National Cancer Institute* 86 (July 6): 955–956.

## 7. Advances in Tumor Imaging

Giger, M. L., and H. MacMahon. In press. Image processing and computer-aided diagnosis. In *Radiologic Clinics of North America*, eds., R. A. Greenes and R. Bauman.

Höhne, K.H., et al, eds. 1991. 3D imaging in medicine. New York: Springer-Verlag.

Udupa, Jayarm K., and Gabor T. Herman. 1991. 3D imaging in medicine. Boca Raton, Fla.: CRC Press.

Vyborny, C. J., and M. L. Giger. 1994. Computer vision and artificial intelligence in mammography. *Journal of Roentgenology* 162 (March): 699–708.

## 8. Advancing Current Treatments for Cancer

DeVita, V. T., Jr., S. Hellman and S. A. Rothenberg eds. 1993. *Cancer: Principles and practice of oncology*, 4th ed. Philadelphia: J. B. Lippincott.

DeVita, V. T., Jr., S. Hellman and S. A. Rothenberg,, eds. 1995. *Biologic therapy of cancer*, 2nd ed. Philadelphia: J. B. Lippincott.

Kartner, Norbert, and Victor Ling. 1989. Multidrug resistance in cancer. *Scientific American* 260 (March): 44–51.

Fact Sheet: Twelve Major Cancers 1996. *The Cancer Journal* 2 (May/June): Supplement.

Murphy, Gerald P., Walter Lawrence, Jr., and Raymond E. Lenhard, Jr. 1995. *American Cancer Society Textbook of Clinical Oncology*, 2nd ed. Atlanta, Ga.: American Cancer Society.

## 9. Immunotherapy for Cancer

Boon, T., et al. 1994. Tumor antigens recognized by T lymphocytes. In *Annual Review of Immunology* 12: 337–366, eds. by W. E. Paul, C. G. Fathman and H. Metzger.

DeVita, V. T., Jr., et al., eds. 1994. *Biologic therapy of cancer*. Philadelphia: Lippincott-Raven.

Goldberg, David M., ed. 1995. *Cancer therapy with radiolabeled antibodies*. Boca Raton, Fla.: CRC Press.

Mach, J. P. 1995. Monoclonal antibodies. In *Oxford Textbook of oncology*, vol. 1, eds., J. Peckham, M. Pindo and U. Veronesi. New York: Oxford University Press.

Sahin, U., et al. 1995. Human neoplasms elicit multiple specific immune responses in the autologous host. *Proceedings of the National Academy of Sciences USA* 92 (December 5): 11810–11813.

## 10. New Molecular Targets for Cancer Therapy

Bishop, J. Michael. 1991. Molecular themes in oncogenesis. *Cell* 64 (January 25): 235–248.

Boguski, Mark S., and Frank McCormick. 1993. Proteins regulating Ras and its relatives. *Nature* 366 (December 16): 643–654.

Gibbs, J. B., and A. Oliff. 1994. Pharmaceutical research in molecular oncology. *Cell* 79 (October 21): 193–198.

Hartwell, Leland H., and Michael B. Kasten. Cell cycle control and cancer. *Science* 266 (December 16): 1821–1828.

Hinds, P. W., and R. A. Weinberg. 1994. Tumor suppressor genes. *Current Opinion in Genetics and Development* 4 (February): 135–141.

## 11. Fighting Cancer by Attacking Its Blood Supply

Folkman, Judah. 1995. Tumor angiogenesis. In *The molecular basis of cancer*, eds., J. Mendelsohn, P.

M. Howley, M. A. Israel and L. A. Liotta. Philadelphia: W. B. Saunders.

Jain, Rakesh K. 1994. Barriers to drug delivery in solid tumors. *Scientific American* 271 (July): 58–65.

O'Reilly, M. S., L. Holmgren, C. Chen and J. Folkman. 1996. Angiostatin induces and sustains dormancy of human primary tumors in mice. *Nature Medicine* 2 (June): 689–692.

Teicher, B. A., N. Dupis, T. Kusomoto, M. F. Robinson, F. Liu, K. Menon and C. N. Coleman. Antiangiogenic agents can increase tumor oxygenation and response to radiation therapy. *Radiation Oncology Investigations* 2: 269–276.

## 12. Cancer's Psychological Challenges

Holland, Jimmie C., and S. Lewis. 1993. Emotions and cancer: What do we really know? In *Mind body medicine: How to use your mind for better health*, eds., Daniel Goleman and Joel Gurin. Yonkers, N.Y.: Consumer Reports Books.

Holland, Jimmie C., and Julia H. Rowland, eds. 1989. *Handbook of psychooncology.* New York: Oxford University Press.

Morra, Marion, and Eve Potts. 1994. *Choices*, 2nd ed. New York: Avon Books.

## 13. Alternative Cancer Treatments

American Cancer Society. 1993. Questionable methods of cancer management: "Nutritional" therapies. *CA Cancer Journal for Clinicians.* 43 (September-October): 309–319.

Brigden, Malcolm L. 1995. Unproven (questionable) cancer therapies. *Western Journal of Medicine* 163 (November): 463–469.

U.S. Congress, Office of Technology Assessment. 1990. *Unconventional cancer treatments*, OTA-H-405. Washington, D.C.: Government Printing Office.

## 14. Controlling the Pain of Cancer

Agency for Health Care Policy and Research. 1994. *Management of cancer pain: Adults.* AHCPR publication No. 94-0593.

Chapman, C. R., and K. M. Foley, eds. 1993. *Current and emerging issues in cancer pain: Research and practice.* Philadelphia: Raven Press.

Melzack, Ronald. 1990. The tragedy of needless pain. *Scientific American* 262 (February): 27–33.

National Cancer Institute. 1995. *Questions and answers about pain control.* NIH publication No. 95-3264.

# Sources of the Photographs

· · ·

Photo Researchers, Inc.: Parts I, II, III, IV, V and VI openings

Merryn MacVille and Thomas Reid, National Center for Human Genome Research, NIH: Figure 1.4

Nina Berman, S/PA: Figure 3.1
EM Unit, CVL Weybridge, Science Photo Library/ Photo Researchers, Inc.: "Papillomavirus"

Jim Lukoski, Black Star: Figure 4.1

Eli Reichman: Figure 6.1
AP/World Wide Photos: "Hubert H. Humphrey"
Johns Hopkins University: "*p53* gene radiograph"

Charles A. Pelizzari: Figures 7.1 and 7.2
Maryellen L. Giger: Figure 7.3

Varian Oncology Systems: "Clinical Linear Accelerators"
Samuel Hellman: "Conformal Radiotherapy"
Mayo Clinic: Figure 8.1
Medtronic, Inc.: Figure 8.2

Varian Associates, Inc.: "Health Workers"
J. Kirk Condyles, Impact Vistas: "Skin Cancer Checkup"
Gina Iannacchero, Dana-Farber Cancer Institute: "Patients"
Jason Goltz: "Use of Taxol"

Pilar Garin-Chesa, Memorial Sloan-Kettering Cancer Center: Figure 9.1
Sydney Welt, Memorial Sloan-Kettering Cancer Center: Figure 9.2
Mark S. Kaminski, University of Michigan: Figure 9.3
Alexander Knuth, Northwest Hospital, Frankfurt: Figure 9.4

Michael S. O'Reilly and Lars Holmgren, Children's Hospital Medical Center, Harvard Medical School: Figure 11.2

Abraham Menashe: Figure 12.2
Blair Seitz: "The Worried Well"

Dartmouth Hitchcock Medical Center: "Getting Doctors to Listen"

# Index

• • •

Page numbers in *italics* indicate illustrations.